W9-BHW-378

DAVID HANCOCK

THE COMPLETE MEDICAL TOURIST

Your Guide to

Inexpensive Dental Cosmetic and
Medical Surgery Abroad

JOHN BLAKE

Published by John Blake Publishing Ltd,
3, Bramber Court, 2 Bramber Road,
London W14 9PB, England

www.blake.co.uk

First published in paperback in 2006

ISBN 1 84454 201 7

All rights reserved. No part of this publication may be
reproduced, stored in a retrieval system, or in any form or by any
means, without the prior permission in writing of the publisher, nor
be otherwise circulated in any form of binding or cover other than
that in which it is published and without a similar condition
including this condition being imposed on the subsequent publisher.

British Library Cataloguing-in-Publication Data:

A catalogue record for this book is available from the
British Library.

Design by www.envydesign.co.uk

Printed in Great Britain by Creative Print & Design, Wales

1 3 5 7 9 10 8 6 4 2

© Text copyright David Hancock, 2006

Papers used by John Blake Publishing are natural, recyclable
products made from wood grown in sustainable forests.
The manufacturing processes conform to the environmental
regulations of the country of origin.

DISCLAIMER

The information contained in this guide is for the purpose of informing the reader of the facilities for medical tourism that may be available around the world. It is not intended to be used for medical diagnosis or treatment, and should not be relied on to suggest a course of treatment for a particular individual. It should in no way be a substitute for a visit, call, consultation or the advice of a qualified doctor or any other healthcare professional. It must be remembered always to consult with a doctor before embarking on any new treatment or health programme. You should never disregard medical advice or delay in seeking it because of something you have read in this guide. All surgery carries some uncertainty and risk, including the possibility of infection, bleeding, blood clots and adverse reactions to the anaesthesia. All risks can be reduced by choosing a qualified surgeon and closely following his or her advice, both before and after surgery. Because a surgeon, hospital, clinic or company is mentioned in this guide it is in no way meant to be an endorsement of their competence.

David Hancock has been a journalist and writer for more than 30 years working for top papers like the *Daily Mirror* and the *Times*. He is the co-author of best-selling books *Stilks* and *A Fighting Chance*, and decided to write about medical tourism when he fractured his pelvis and learned the bitter lesson of the National Health System at first hand. He lives in Highbury, North London.

*Dedicated to my mother and the memory
of my late father*

ACKNOWLEDGEMENTS

Obviously, a book of this sort means a lot of research, but I would especially like to thank the following organisations for making information available: Medical Tourism.com; Gynaecomastia.org; lipoinfo.com; American Society Of Plastic Surgeons; iEnhance; PlasticSurgery.com; netdoctor.co.uk; Direct Healthcare International; Wikipedia.org; Surgeon & Safari; RS Cosmetic Clinic.

If you or your company are involved in the area of medical tourism and feel you should be included in the next edition of this handbook then please email davidhancockuk@hotmail.com.

INTRODUCTION

Medical tourism is one of the fastest-growing businesses on earth. In less than a decade it has become a worldwide multi-billion-pound industry that has transformed the lives of people all over the globe.

The term 'medical tourist' refers to a person who, for whatever reason, decides to leave their own country and have their medical, surgical or dental treatment performed abroad. Reasons for doing this vary, but usually it comes down to cost. It is simply much cheaper to have medical or cosmetic treatment abroad than it is to have it in the UK, the USA or Canada.

Medical tourism is actually thousands of years old. The ancient Greeks knew all about it and pilgrims would travel from all over the Mediterranean to seek the powers of the healing god Asklepios at Epidaurus. In Roman Britain, the city of Bath was famous for its restorative waters and would attract people from all over the Roman Empire. And in the 18th century, spa towns from Germany to the Nile were the watering-holes for wealthy Europeans.

But now, with the increase in low-cost worldwide air travel, medical tourism is no longer the privilege of the rich elite. It is within the reach of everybody. With the ever-escalating cost of hospital treatment in the UK and the USA, and especially with long waiting lists in the UK for treatment on its overstretched National Health Service, more and more people are looking to other countries for faster and cheaper cures in state-of-the-art environments.

Mass international tourism has made people less resistant or fearful of visiting a hospital and trusting a surgeon abroad because they have become familiar with the country. And once the tourist has seen how much cheaper treatment is abroad and how quickly procedures can be done, it is not surprising that medical tourism is booming. Hip-replacement treatment in Britain using metal-to-metal resurfacing, for instance, can cost £12,000. Take a trip on the Eurostar train through the Channel Tunnel to Belgium, however, and the cost can be slashed down to £6,500. Fly to one of the latest high-tech hospitals in India, which have been specially built to cater for medical tourism, and that same operation, performed by doctors trained in the West, falls to only £3,700.

And it is not just cost that has become a deciding factor in medical tourism. The threat of killer superbugs like MRSA, which have become rife in some British hospitals in recent years, are also playing a part. In most worldwide hospitals these superbugs are found in much smaller numbers.

Add to that spotless private hospital rooms, one-to-one nursing care and food often cooked by top qualified chefs and the argument for medical tourism starts to become irresistible. So irresistible, in fact, that the British government has even begun sending patients abroad in an effort to cut the backlog of people waiting for an operation on the NHS.

When you realise that post-operative convalescence can take place in a top-class hotel in a warm holiday destination, and everything can be arranged in advance, it's something worth thinking about. Many people combine their medical treatment with a couple of weeks of sightseeing.

The growth in cheap worldwide travel means that no destination is really out of reach of the discerning medical tourist. The more exotic places like South America, Thailand and India have seen the greatest influx in medical tourism. A bone marrow transplant in the USA could cost a staggering £140,000 but you can get the operation done in Mumbai, formerly Bombay, in India for only £26,000 – a fraction of the cost. But it is not just countries with sun-drenched beaches that have become appealing. In Abbeville in northern France, less than an hour from the port of Calais, is a state-of-the-art modern hospital that caters almost entirely for British patients.

As medical tourism grows so does the variety of operations provided. Whether it is elective cosmetic surgery like liposuction or rhinoplasty, or a more serious procedure such as a heart bypass, they can all be carried out abroad at a portion of the cost at home.

Many countries now actively promote medical tourism as part of their economy, chief among them being India where it is estimated the industry will grow by 30 per cent a year and account for £1 billion in earnings by 2012. So keen is the Indian government on medical tourism that the country's National Health Policy has deemed it to be legally an 'export' and 'eligible for all fiscal incentives extended to export earnings'. Special hospitals have been built on the subcontinent and there are half a dozen specialist medical corporations catering for the new industry. The largest is Apollo Hospital Enterprises, which treated an estimated 60,000 patients between 2001 and spring 2004. Apollo now has 37 hospitals with about 7,000 beds.

Thailand is another country at the forefront of medical tourism, with Bangkok's International Medical Centre offering services in 26 languages. Other countries actively promoting the new industry include Hungary, Costa Rica, Israel, Belgium, Poland, Malaysia and South Africa.

But it's a jungle out there, and the last thing any would-be patient wants to do is spend hours and hours trying to find the best service available. So we have done that for you. In this book you will find information on locations, hospitals, procedures and sightseeing. It should be borne in mind that any prices quoted in this guide are an approximation only because costs can change due either to inflation or fluctuations in currency.

Always remember: just because you have had treatment and a holiday abroad don't think it will be some sort of catch-all cure for any medical condition, or that you will simply be able to get up and walk away with no after effects. Don't think you will be able to spring back into health after you come round from the anaesthetic just because you had the operation overseas.

All the same rules apply as if you had been operated on in Britain. Back in the UK you would have had to have gone through a period of rehabilitation. This is especially true with major surgery such as transplants where, even after a significant period of recuperation, you will have to go on to take drugs daily for the rest of your life.

With orthopaedic surgery, especially hip and knee replacements, you will need to undertake a fairly lengthy period of physiotherapy once you are back home.

So remember to inform your GP of any surgery you are thinking of having before you go abroad. The GP will not only be able to advise you on side-effects and the length of recuperation back in the UK but also help arrange any rehabilitation you may need.

CONTENTS

SECTION ONE

Chapter One

CARDIAC SURGERY

Coronary heart disease claimed the lives of 233,000 people in the UK in 2003, according to the British Heart Foundation. More than 1.4 million people suffer from angina and 260,000 people had a heart attack in the UK in 2003. These are astonishing statistics, making coronary heart disease the biggest killer in the country.

In order to work properly the heart needs a constant supply of oxygen, which is carried in the blood and flows through the heart's blood vessels. When the supply is blocked or interrupted due to a build-up of fatty substances in the arteries, heart disease occurs. A partial blocking can lead to angina, the symptoms of which are chest pains. A complete blockage leads to a heart attack.

A combination of regular exercise with a change to a low-fat diet with a lower salt intake and more fresh fruit, oily fish, vegetables and cereals can help the prevention of heart disease by increasing the level of HDL cholesterol (the good cholesterol). Needless to say, smokers should stop smoking, as it hardens the arteries and causes the majority of cases of coronary thrombosis in people under the age of 50.

HEART BYPASS

The most effective form of treatment for people with hardened and narrowed arteries is the heart bypass, although contrary to popular opinion it is best in those who have *not* had a heart attack and whose heart is not enlarged.

The two coronary arteries come off the main artery of the body, the aorta. The left coronary artery immediately divides into two, so there are three main coronary branches. If necessary, a bypass can be done on all three. This is called a triple bypass. Veins stripped from the leg were almost always used to make the bypass. They were connected to the coronary arteries beyond the narrowed areas and then linked to the aorta, just above the heart. But in recent years surgeons have been preferring to connect an internal artery of the chest wall to the diseased coronary artery. This means that the surgeon can use keyhole surgery, which is minimally invasive, and the heart does not have to be stopped during the operation. Small plastic devices, known as stents, are used to keep the arteries open.

Bypass surgery, performed under general anaesthetic, takes between three and six hours after which there is a period in an intensive care unit. Within two days of surgery, you should be able to sit out of bed and, if you have an office job, be able to return to it within six weeks. More demanding manual work may mean three months off, and patients are advised not to drive for at least a month after the surgery.

Although heart-bypass surgery is major, it is very common and quite safe with less than a 2 per cent risk to life. Most patients get another 10 years free of heart symptoms but they need to change their lifestyle as well. Regular exercise, stopping smoking and a healthier diet are all good advice.

UK cost (approx): £12,000–15,000
See Section Two: Belgium; Germany; India; Malaysia;
                    South Africa

MITRAL-VALVE OPERATION

The mitral valve is the inflow valve for the left-hand side of the heart, allowing blood to flow into the heart's main pumping chamber, and closing to prevent the blood from going back into the lungs before it has been pumped around the body. As we age, the mitral valve can degenerate, or it may be damaged by infection or rheumatic fever. They can also be affected by heart attacks or congenitally. Sometimes the mitral valve has to be replaced, but it can often be repaired.

In replacement surgery, the valve is made usually from titanium; this lasts forever but the patient has to be given blood thinners for the remainder of his or her life. A valve can also be made from a cow or pig's heart;

the patient doesn't need anticoagulation treatment, but these valves do wear out after about 12 to 15 years.

During the operation, under general anaesthetic, the patient is connected to a heart and lung machine, which takes over from the patient's real heart and lungs while the surgeon opens up the heart to see whether the mitral valve is damaged and can be repaired or whether it has to be replaced. After the operation, patients are transferred to a special unit for open-heart cases before draining catheters are taken out and they can return to a normal hospital room. Hospitalisation usually takes about seven days.

The future of mitral-valve operations is with minimally invasive videoscopic and robotic techniques, where the only incision needed is merely two-and-a-half inches long.

Heart-valve-repair operations take between three and five hours and full recovery can take a few months. An exercise programme is often recommended along with a lifestyle change of diet, and an awareness that valves sometimes have to be replaced.

UK cost (approx): £10,000+
See Section Two: Belgium; Germany; India; South
                   Africa

ANGIOGRAM

Doctors can tell how well blood moves through the vessels of your body by taking an angiogram, which is really an X-ray examination of those blood vessels. A coronary angiogram is done by inserting a small tube through the skin into the artery, guiding it to the opening of the coronary arteries and injecting a dye (usually a solution of iodine) which can be traced by X-ray pictures. The images are called the angiogram and can reveal the extent and severity of any artery blockages or narrowing.

The procedure – performed with local anaesthetic – usually takes about 30 minutes and is not terribly uncomfortable; the insertion is either through the arm or the groin.

UK cost (approx): £1,000–3,160
See Section Two: Belgium; Germany; India;
South Africa

BALLOON DILATION

Fat and cholesterol that has formed on the inside of arteries is known as plaque. If the narrowing or blocking of the arteries due to plaque is not too severe, then the artery can be opened using a balloon catheter as an alternative to bypass surgery. The inflated balloon widens the blocked vessel and restores adequate blood supply. The artery is kept open by placing a stent at the site of the blockage and the whole procedure is known as an angioplasty.

Although this procedure treats the condition, it does not cure the cause and narrowing may or may not reoccur. Patients are often post-operatively treated with blood thinners as well as statins to lower cholesterol, and advised to change their lifestyle patterns with a healthier diet, exercise and stopping smoking.

The average hospital stay for the procedure is two days and complete recovery takes a week or less, with patients able to walk within six hours of the operation.

UK cost (approx): £11,600–15,000
See Section Two: Belgium; Germany; India;
                   South Africa

Chapter Two

COSMETIC SURGERY

More and more people are deciding to change the way they look by having cosmetic surgery. And, in line with the increase in demand, there have been major advances in these kinds of elective procedures. It is no longer just the rich or the celebrity-conscious who are having their bodies resculptured; prices have now become so affordable that anyone who can take a holiday can afford a little nip and tuck.

In the age group of 18 or younger, the dominant procedure is ear surgery; breast augmentation is popular with women aged 19–35, while the over-50s go for eyelid surgery or facelifts.

For many years, it was assumed that only women took advantage of cosmetic surgery, but that has all changed. Today, more men than ever are aware of the way they look, and just as a whole industry of male facial creams, scrubs, lotions and other cosmetics has built up, so has the desire in men to change their appearance. For many, it is a greater awareness of health issues as mirrored in the growth of men's magazines. For others, it is the intense competition in the business world. The perception, correct or not, is that an older man is less up-to-date and efficient. So in an effort to remain looking young many men are turning to cosmetic surgery. And there are some operations that are peculiar only to men, such as treatment for gynaecomastia (large breasts), penile surgery and hair transplants.

But, male or female, before embarking on any form of cosmetic enhancement read as much as you can about your chosen procedure or treatment. This will help you to make sure it is right for you and you are aware of the pros and cons of the treatment. Be clear about what you want to achieve. Find out all you can about the doctor who will be performing the surgery and, at an initial consultation, don't be afraid to ask the surgeon about his or her qualifications and expertise in the procedure. Ask how many times they have performed the operation and whether complications have ever occurred. Choose the clinic or hospital carefully by reading as much literature as possible so you can compare prices and services. Don't ignore the risks – all surgery can have risks.

This guide is an excellent starting point for that research.

BREAST REDUCTION

Breast size is determined by genes, hormones, weight and body frame and for most women the breast size is in proportion to their frame. But when it is not it can cause both psychological distress and physical discomfort. For some women, large breasts can develop in adolescence because of the hormone oestrogen, and for others it may happen later in life following the menopause or use of Hormone Replacement Therapy. Either way, it can be distressing for women, leaving them with an overbearing feeling of self-consciousness. Some women may even have breasts of a different size or shape and in these circumstances surgery may be undertaken to reduce the larger one. But it must be emphasised that breast reduction is not vital for one's health and so for this reason it is classified as cosmetic surgery, even though there is some evidence that breast reduction may decrease the chances of developing breast cancer (according to Bandolier, 2001).

Although excessively large breasts, known medically as mammary hypertrophy, may not be life-threatening, they can cause distressing problems like back and neck strain, poor posture and shortness of breath, and can be both socially and sexually embarrassing. Women with pendulous breasts may also find difficulty in buying clothes due to the disproportion, and many become so self-conscious that they try to camouflage their body shape by wearing baggy clothing, avoiding recreational activities and in extreme cases become introverted, reclusive and depressed.

Normally, a female breast reduction will take a surgeon about three hours and will be carried out under general anaesthetic. The patient will be expected to stay in hospital overnight. The operation involves reducing and uplifting the breast tissue at the same time. Techniques vary but usually involve an anchor-shaped incision that circles the areola, extends downwards and follows the natural curve of the crease beneath the breast. Excess glandular tissue, fat and skin are removed and the nipple and areola moved into their new position. The movement of the nipple carries with it the risk that the woman may not be able to breastfeed after surgery.

Modern surgical techniques, especially using liposuction, mean breast reduction can leave minimal scarring. After surgery, the breasts are wrapped in an elastic bandage or surgical bra over gauze dressings, and pain may be experienced for the first few days. The first menstruation following surgery may also cause the breasts to swell and hurt.

Patients are advised to take things easy and not return to work for at least two weeks after surgery. As a medical tourist, it is the time to relax and enjoy being pampered. Although the swelling and bruising will disappear before it is time to return home, it may take six months to a year before the breasts settle into their new shape, so patience is required.

No surgery is without risks, although these can be greatly lessened by taking the advice of the surgeon to make sure the patient is in good health before the operation. Side-effects specific to breast reduction may include losing sensation in the nipple and experiencing scarring, which usually takes quite some time to fade. The new breasts may also feel tender and lumpy for some weeks or even months after the procedure.

UK cost (approx): £4,550–5,600
See Section Two: Argentina; Belgium; Czech
                   Republic; Egypt; Germany; Greece;
                   Hungary; India; Mexico; Poland;
                   South Africa; Spain; Thailand;
                   Tunisia; Turkey

GYNAECOMASTIA

For obvious reasons, men with abnormally large breasts can be left with feelings of shame and embarrassment, and it can leave sufferers with deeper psychological issues to deal with than those of women with large breasts. A man or boy with gynaecomastia struggles with anxiety over such simple acts as taking off his shirt at the beach. The condition is relatively common in adolescent boys, and 90 per cent of the time symptoms disappear in a matter of months or, as adolescence wanes, a few years later. But the remaining 10 per cent are burdened with a social handicap that causes a deep and complex shame, and puts one's relationship with one's body at risk.

There are many reasons for the development of gynaecomastia, from a genetic disorder which occurs at conception known as Klinefelter Syndrome, in which the chromosomes in the sex line have at least one extra 'X', to the abuse of steroids by bodybuilders, often known as 'bitch tits'. The ageing process itself in men can also cause gynaecomastia. But the men who suffer the greatest problems are those who have been aware of the condition since adolescence and have tried to hide it.

Surgery can help, though it is not the preferred option and is discouraged in men who are overweight and have not attempted to correct the problem with exercise and weight loss. Excess breast tissue is removed through an incision around the nipple and the procedure can be done in two hours under general anaesthetic, requiring no overnight stay in hospital. After surgery, the patient is fitted with a compression garment or ace bandages to support the breasts while they heal.

Considering the amount of emotional damage that gynaecomastia can cause to a sufferer, a surgical solution is relatively quick and patients can be back to work within seven days, although bruising, numbness and soreness will last longer. Any complications usually only stem from surgeon error or the patient trying to do too much after the operation.

UK cost (approx): £1,800–4,750
See Section Two: Argentina; Belgium; Egypt; Greece; India; Mexico; Poland; South Africa; Spain; Thailand; Tunisia; Turkey

LIPOSUCTION

Contrary to popular belief, very obese people are not really suitable for liposuction, which is the removal of excess fatty tissue to reshape the body. Instead, they should diet and exercise first. Liposuction is aimed at getting rid of the stubborn fat left after diet and exercise. In women, the most frequently treated areas are the abdomen, hips, thighs and knees, and in men it is love handles, abdomen, arms, neck and face. Sweat glands in the underarm can also be removed by liposuction without it affecting the body's ability to cool itself.

Liposuction was invented in Rome as far back as 1974 by Dr Giorgio Fischer. It has been constantly developed and refined, and now there are different methods employed – from the tumescent technique, which uses large volumes of lightly salted water solution, to standard liposuction methods, which require a general anaesthetic. A more modern technique uses ultrasonic energy to explode the walls of fat cells.

With standard liposuction, the patient is given a general anaesthetic and the surgeon uses a hand-held instrument called a cannula, which might be partly or completely made of metal or plastic, to suck out the fat. The fat is pulled out into a suction machine. In order for the liposuction treatment to be long lasting, the patient must stick to a proper diet and exercise plan after the operation.

The method of liposuction used depends on patient and surgeon preference, and anyone considering undergoing the treatment is advised to find out about all types, and which methods certain surgeons use. It is claimed by some specialists that recovery and return to work and daily functions are faster following tumescent liposuction as opposed to traditional/standard liposuction, with significant numbing lasting only 18 hours in the suctioned areas. The post-operative recovery period is also claimed to be only one or two days, allowing for a longer holiday while abroad.

However, like any surgery, it carries risks, which include infection, blood clots, nerve damage and numbness.

Side-effects in all methods of liposuction include bruising, soreness and swelling, but these should disappear completely within a few weeks.

UK cost (approx): £2,000–5,150
See Section Two: Argentina; Belgium; Czech
                   Republic; Egypt; Germany;
                   Hungary; India; Italy; Malaysia;
                   Mexico; Poland; South Africa;
                   Spain; Thailand; Tunisia; Turkey

BREAST ENLARGEMENT

Thanks to the high profile of stars like Pamela Anderson and Jordan, breast enlargements are on a par with facelifts as the best-known cosmetic surgery procedures. Unfortunately, it has also led many young women to believe that all that's needed to achieve fame and fortune is a quick breast augmentation. Of course, nothing could be further from the truth.

So the first thing to do before embarking on this course of treatment is to ask yourself honestly why you want it done. And there are plenty of good reasons why. A loss of breast volume after pregnancy; difference in size between the two breasts; breast size that has reduced after losing weight; or simply a feeling that they are too small or out of proportion. Breast enlargement, or augmentation mammoplasty to give it its technical term, can enhance appearance and self-confidence but is ideally for women looking for improvement, not perfection.

Modern implants are usually made from a special cohesive silicon filling which makes them less likely to leak than the silicone in older implants, and they are inserted through incisions on or near the breasts. The exact position varies. It can be around the nipple, towards the armpit, or in the crease under the breast. Once the implant is in place, the incision is closed with stitches and bandages or dressings applied to the wound. The procedure is usually done under general anaesthetic, taking between one and two hours, and is most likely performed as a day case without needing an overnight stay in hospital.

Breast augmentation is relatively straightforward and the vast majority of women have no problems whatsoever. Some pain and bruising occurs around the breasts for the first few days, but this can be controlled by painkillers and wearing a special supporting bra following surgery.

Some women report that their nipples become oversensitive, undersensitive or even numb, but this usually passes with time. There is no evidence that breast implants cause breast cancer but they can change the way mammography is done to detect cancer. Additional views may be required by the X-ray technician and ultrasound examinations may also be of benefit. There is also no evidence that implants will affect fertility or pregnancy. The major worry for most women is whether the implant will break or leak as a result of injury or normal compression and movement. But, while this problem is uncommon with modern implants, anyone considering this type of surgery should be aware of what could happen. If a saline-filled implant breaks, the implant will deflate and the salt water will be absorbed harmlessly by the body. In the case of a gel-filled implant, the woman may not detect any change if the shell breaks but the capsule around the implant does not. But, if the capsule also breaks, gel may move into surrounding tissue or migrate to another area of the body. In both cases, a second operation and replacement of the leaking implant will be necessary.

The most common problem is that the capsule around the implant begins to contract and tighten, squeezing the soft implant and making the breasts feel hard. This can be treated, usually by a replacement of the implant.

Patients should be able to shower about four days after

the operation and, within a week, any stitches that are not dissolvable are taken out. Within a few weeks, the breasts will settle into their new shape, and for many women the results can be very satisfying as they appreciate their new appearance. But remember that over time even breasts with implants will begin to sag and further surgery to lift the breasts may have to be considered.

UK cost (approx): £4,050–4,650
See Section Two: Argentina; Belgium; Czech
                 Republic; Egypt; Germany; Greece;
                 Hungary; India; Malaysia; Mexico;
                 Poland;
                 South Africa; Spain; Thailand;
                 Tunisia; Turkey

TUMMY TUCK

This is a major surgical technique also known as abdominoplasty, which removes excess skin and fat from the middle and lower abdomen to tighten the muscles of the abdominal wall. It can work wonders for people who are left with folds of loose skin or large fat deposits that won't respond to diet and exercise. It is especially good for women who have stretched their abdominal muscles and lost skin elasticity through multiple pregnancies. But anyone electing to have the procedure must remember that it does leave a permanent scar, which, depending on the size of the operation, can extend from hip to hip.

There are several different tummy-tuck techniques. The most common procedure is performed under general anaesthetic. In the full tummy tuck, an incision is made across the lower abdomen, just above the pubic area. Another incision is made around the belly button to free the surrounding skin, and all of the skin is separated from the abdominal wall. Then the surgeon pulls the loose muscles from the left and the right sides and stitches them together. This tightens the muscles to create a stronger abdominal wall and a smaller waist. Excess skin is removed, and a new opening is made for the belly button at the right position. The incisions are closed with stitches and staples, and gauze is placed over the incision area.

A full tuck usually takes between two and five hours, and most people stay in hospital for one to three days after the procedure. For the first few days, the patient will be asked to keep their knees and hips bent while they sleep at night to reduce strain on the stitches. Stitches in the skin will normally be removed in five to seven days and deeper stitches closing the operation site may be taken out two to three weeks after surgery. It may take several weeks to feel completely back to normal. If the patient is in top physical condition, recovery will be much faster. Some people return to work after two weeks, while others take four weeks to recuperate.

Even if the patient has never exercised before, they should begin a light exercise programme to reduce swelling, lower the chance of blood clots and improve muscle tone. However, vigorous exercise, especially lifting, should be postponed until it can be done comfortably and the doctor has given permission. Scars may appear to worsen during the first few months, but this is normal. It may take up to a year before the scars flatten out and lighten in colour. While they'll never disappear completely, these scars will be placed so that they'll be covered by clothes, including most bathing costumes.

Many people who believe they need a tummy tuck may in fact need only liposuction, and a surgeon will give advice on the best procedure. Regardless of which is chosen, it is best for a patient to get their weight down as much as possible before deciding on medical treatment.

If the only problem area is below the belly button, a person may benefit from a less complex procedure called a partial abdominoplasty or partial tummy tuck, which can often be performed on an outpatient basis, under local anaesthetic such as that used by dentists.

UK cost (approx): £4,250–5,370
See Section Two: Argentina; Belgium; Czech
                   Republic; Egypt; Germany;
                   Hungary; India; Mexico;
                   South Africa; Spain; Thailand;
                   Tunisia; Turkey

FACELIFT

The mother of all cosmetic surgery is the rhytidectomy. The face is without a doubt the most prominent physical feature of all human beings. Every morning we get up and look at it, wash it, women make it up with powder and paint, men shave it, we examine it, stare at it and, above all, shallow or not, it is why other people are initially attracted to us and what makes them fall in love. The face rules.

A facelift is completely elective cosmetic surgery with no medical reasons for the treatment, but it can conceal age, restore youthful appearance and therefore boost confidence. More than 90 per cent of all facelifts are performed on women, but in recent years it has started to become more popular with men. And in Brazil, where facelifts are *de rigueur*, veterinary surgeons even perform them on dogs to straighten bent ears or use Botox to fix inverted eyelashes. A few years ago, an award-winning Pekingese in Britain was the subject of an inquiry when rumours swirled that its face had been surgically enhanced. The dog and its owners were acquitted and allowed to keep the award from the 2003 Crufts Dog Show.

Although rhytidectomy is from the Greek meaning 'removal of wrinkles', not all wrinkles are eradicated with a facelift. Those around the mouth and eyes, for instance, may benefit little, and other treatments, such as a chemical peel or dermabrasion, may be necessary. So it is important to know the limits of a facelift before deciding to have one. This will depend on the bone structure of your face and should be discussed with your cosmetic surgeon, who will know the amount of treatment to be given.

Preparation is necessary for a good facelift. If, for instance, you colour your hair, do so before having surgery, as you can't use hair dye for four to six weeks after treatment. Avoid pills that contain aspirin as these thin the blood, and a good facelift depends on excellent blood clotting.

The surgery will last between four and six hours and can be performed with a mixture of local and 'twilight' anaesthetics, which help lower the awareness of the procedure. It is not recommended that you have only local anaesthetic because you will then be awake during the procedure. Many patients who are awake are squirmy and remember the surgery.

There are many variations of facelift surgery but in a typical version the surgeon begins by making an incision within the hairline just above the ear. The incision continues down along the front edge of the ear, around the earlobe and then up and behind the ear extending back into the hairline. The location of this incision is designed to hide any sign of the procedure later. The same procedure is repeated on the other side of the face. Using various instruments, the surgeon will then work to separate the skin of the face from its underlying tissue, moving down to the cheek and into the neck area and below the chin. Fat deposits over the cheeks and in the neck may be removed surgically or with liposuction at this time. The surgeon will then work to free up and tighten certain bands of muscle and tissue that extend up from the shoulder, below the chin, and up and behind the neck. If these muscles and tissue are not tightened, the looseness and sagging appearance of the skin will return. The surgeon then trims excess skin from the edges of the original incision, pulls the skin back and staples or stitches it into place. Finally, at the end of the procedure, a small tube is placed behind or near the ear where the stitches are located to drain away any fluids, and sterile dressings and bandages are applied to secure the head and neck area and prevent infection.

Many surgeons recommend that patients remain reclining either in their hotel room or at home for the next 24 hours, consume a liquid diet and avoid any movements that need the neck to flex. Ice packs can reduce swelling and antibiotics are taken as a precaution until the first stitches come out after about five days. Many medical tourists return home after a couple of weeks and go back to work and limited activities.

There are risks involved in facelift surgery. The largest risk lies in the possibility that the facelift will not bring the desired results. A facelift can't completely get rid of deep wrinkles or change the structure of a person's face. Skin changes in texture and it will thin over time. Lifts won't change that.

One complication seen following facelift surgery is a haematoma – a mass of clotted blood that forms in a tissue. If a haematoma forms, the patient may need to return and have the stitches reopened to find the source of the bleeding. Most haematomas form within 48 hours of surgery. The typical sign is pain or swelling affecting one side of the face but not the other. Another risk is nerve damage. Sometimes it can affect the patient's ability to raise an eyebrow, or it can distort the smile, or leave the patient with limited feeling in the earlobe. Most of these nerve injuries, however, repair themselves within two to six months.

But most skilled cosmetic surgeons these days can eliminate all risks. The real risk comes if the patient gets hooked on facelift surgery and starts demanding more and more until the skin becomes too tightly stretched – and we have all seen certain celebrities looking like that. The results of a facelift usually last for between five and ten years depending on one's age – the older you are, the shorter the time the results last.

There are alternatives to facelifts that are less drastic. Age-spot removal and tightening can be achieved with forms of laser treatment, and Botox injections can lessen wrinkling in the forehead and outer eye area. Not smoking or drinking alcohol, but exercising, keeping out of the sun, drinking lots of water and moisturising the face will all help to stave off the ageing process.

UK cost (approx): £4,000–9,000
See Section Two: Argentina; Belgium; Czech Republic; Egypt; Germany; Hungary; India; Malaysia; Mexico; Poland; South Africa; Spain; Thailand; Tunisia; Turkey

NOSE RESHAPING

The 'nose job' is one of the most common of all cosmetic surgery procedures. And it's not just people with large noses that want them reshaped. A rhinoplasty procedure can reduce or increase the size of the nose, change the shape of the tip or the bridge, narrow the span of the nostrils, or change the angle between the nose and the upper lip. It may also correct a birth defect or injury, or help relieve some breathing problems.

By the age of 16, your nose is fully developed, and if you want to change it you must be clear in your mind what you dislike about its appearance so that you can tell your surgeon. It's no use simply saying, 'I hate my nose.' The good thing about rhinoplasty is that the overwhelming majority of people are very happy with their nose after surgery and their self-confidence is boosted immeasurably.

The operation, performed under general anaesthetic, is carried out inside the nostrils so that there are no external scars – unless you decide to have the size of the nostrils reduced, in which case small scars around the sides of the nostrils, placed in the natural crease lines between nose and cheek, will be present. The shape of the nose is created by partially removing and reshaping bone and cartilage, with the skin over the nose left untouched. The elasticity of the skin means that it can shrink down to the new shape.

If you are having nose augmentation, the surgeon may need additional bone to build up the nose and this is usually taken from your hip, a rib, the back of your elbow or the surface of your skull. Extra cartilage can be taken from your ears or spare cartilage inside the nose.

A normal nose job takes between one and two hours and a splint may be applied to make sure the nose maintains its new shape. There will be swelling and bruising around the eyes and things may look a lot worse than they feel, but you should be able to enjoy your holiday – although avoid strenuous exercise like swimming or jogging, or anything that might increase your blood pressure. You should also be able to return to work after a two-to-three-week holiday, by which time the swelling and bruising should have disappeared.

You might experience some unexpected reactions from family and friends. They may say they don't see a major difference in your nose. Or they may be resentful, especially if you've changed something they view as a family or ethnic trait. If that happens, try to keep in mind why you decided to have this surgery in the first place. If you've met your goals, then your surgery is a success.

UK cost (approx): £3,200–3,800
See Section Two: Argentina; Belgium; Czech
                   Republic; Egypt; Germany;
                   Hungary; India; Mexico; Poland;
                   South Africa; Spain; Thailand;
                   Tunisia; Turkey

EYE–BAG REMOVAL

If you have ever looked in the mirror and thought, 'Who's that Doberman?' then it might be time for a little blepharoplasty – or eye-bag removal.

The hound-dog look makes you appear older and more tired than you feel, and in some cases can even interfere with your vision. This surgical procedure removes fat along with excess skin and muscle from the upper and lower eyelids. What it doesn't do is remove crow's feet and other wrinkles, or lift sagging eyebrows. But a blepharoplasty is often done in conjunction with other procedures such as a facelift or brow-lift, and is usually performed on middle-aged or older people using local anaesthetic – which numbs the area around the eyes – along with oral or intravenous sedatives. You'll be awake during the surgery, but relaxed and insensitive to pain. The typical eyelid surgery involves the plastic surgeon making incisions within the natural lines of the eyelids. These surgical incisions are placed within the creases of the upper eyelids and directly below the eyelashes in the lower lids. Once these incisions are made, the surgeon separates the skin and removes the excess fat, tissue and muscle. Following the removal of all excess tissues, the incisions are stitched together in an effort to expedite the healing process.

In those blepharoplasty cases where lower-eyelid fat is being removed, but no skin is being displaced, the plastic surgeon may elect to use a technique referred to as a transconjunctival blepharoplasty. In this procedure, the surgical incision is placed within the interior of the lower eyelid, resulting in no visible scar.

Because the eyes are the focal point on the face, upper-eyelid blepharoplasty may achieve anything from a subtle to a dramatic improvement in a person's appearance. For this, and such reasons as its relatively modest cost and quick recovery, many people choose blepharoplasty over a full facelift.

After surgery, the surgeon will probably lubricate your eyes with ointment and may apply a bandage. Your eyelids may feel tight and sore as the anaesthetic wears off, and you may be instructed to keep your head elevated for several days and use cold compresses to reduce swelling and bruising. You should be able to read or watch television after two or three days, and most people feel ready to go out in public in a week. By then, depending on your rate of healing and your doctor's instructions, you'll probably be able to wear makeup to hide the bruising that remains. You may be sensitive to sunlight, wind and other irritants for several weeks, so you should wear sunglasses and a special sunblock made for eyelids when you go out. You should also avoid bending over, wearing contact lenses and driving until healed.

The positive results of eyelid surgery, making you look more youthful and alert, last for years.

UK cost (approx):   Lower eyelids £2,080–3,100; upper eyelids £2,150–3,300; upper and lower eyelids £3,000–4,325

See Section Two: Argentina; Belgium; Czech Republic; Egypt; Germany; Hungary; India; Mexico; Poland; South Africa; Spain; Thailand; Tunisia; Turkey

BREAST UPLIFT

Pregnancy, nursing babies and the force of gravity eventually take their toll on a woman's breasts. And, as the skin loses its elasticity, the breasts lose their shape, their firmness, and begin to sag and point to the floor rather than the opposite wall. A mastopexy is a procedure to raise and reshape sagging breasts – at least for a time – before gravity comes into play again.

The best results are usually achieved in women with small sagging breasts and may last longer than those in women with heavier breasts, but breasts of any size can be lifted. The treatment is done under general anaesthetic. It can take between one and four hours, and there are three basic types of technique.

During concentric mastopexy, circular incisions are made around the areola. The skin between the two incisions, shaped something like a doughnut, is removed, the nipple and areola is replaced, usually moved upwards, and the surrounding skin is stitched to the skin around the areola. Because there is a relatively small amount of skin removal, this technique will only work for women with smaller breasts and minimal sagging.

In vertical mastopexy, using a similar technique to that of concentric mastopexy, the surgeon will extend the incision vertically below the areola to the breast crease by the chest. This approach allows an additional strip of skin to be removed, giving the surgeon the option of greater correction.

Finally, there is the anchor-shaped mastopexy, the most invasive and most common type of breast-lift surgery. An incision is made above the nipple in the shape of an anchor, with a circle at the top. This incision forms the shape of the new breast with the nipple placed in the circle at the top of the anchor, and the elliptical line at the bottom forming the lower contour. After the incision, the skin below is removed, the breast tissue and nipple lifted to a higher position, and the incision site is stitched closed.

After surgery, you'll wear an elastic bandage or a surgical bra over gauze dressings. Your breasts will be bruised, swollen and uncomfortable for a day or two, but the pain shouldn't be severe. The surgical bra will be worn from between one and two weeks and after that a well-fitting sports bra should be worn for four to six weeks. Any numbness will subside, although it may take some time, and in extreme cases can last more than six months. Women who have an implant at the same time as an uplift usually find that the uplift lasts longer, even as nature takes it course.

UK cost (approx): £3,800–4,850

See Section Two: Argentina; Belgium; Czech
Republic; Egypt; Germany;
Hungary; India; Mexico; Poland;
South Africa; Spain; Thailand;
Tunisia; Turkey

PENIS ENLARGEMENT

It's an age-old question: does penis size matter? And the answer is: only if it matters to the man in question. Research shows that penis size does not affect partner satisfaction during sexual intercourse, even if the penis is severely shortened to less than 5 centimetres (2 inches), and women are more likely to be bemused by men's obsession with the size of their manhood than amused by its smallness.

Yet for many men the size of their penis can fill them with an anxiety that dogs them throughout their life and causes them to question their masculinity. One of the reasons for this is that some men have a short, fat, rather elastic penis when soft that expands considerably when erect, while other men have long, flaccid penises that barely lengthen when rigid. When men from the first group see men from the second group naked in the showers at the gym or swimming pool for instance, they often automatically think they are deficient in some way. Both are normal, just different. The famous Masters and Johnson survey of 1966 found that the length of an erect penis varied from 12.5 centimetres (5 inches) to 17.5

centimetres (7 inches) with 12.9 centimetres (5.2 inches) being the average. A penis enlargement, or penile augmentation, is recommended only for those with a flaccid length of less than 4 centimetres (1.6 inches) or an erect length of less than 7.5 centimetres (3 inches).

While private clinics around the world may make extravagant claims about penis-enlargement surgery, the jury is still out on whether it works or can be of any benefit at all. The procedures are largely unproven by research; many urologists consider the surgery to be experimental and may carry the risk of serious complications. For this reason, many top cosmetic surgeons refuse to carry out penis-enlargement procedures.

Among those that do, there are several techniques involved. One technique for lengthening is to cut the suspensory ligament, which has the role of keeping the penis pointing upwards during erection. Plastic surgery is then used to provide additional skin to cover the new length. The only reliable study available on this technique indicates that the maximum length gain is around 1.6 centimetres (0.75 inches) in the flaccid state, while the erect penis is about the same size but now points to the floor.

A technique to increase the thickness, or girth, of the penis includes injecting liposuctioned fat from the thighs into the penile shaft, or grafting tissue and fat on to the penis. Grafts seem to do better than liposuctioned fat, 90 per cent of which can disappear within a year.

There can be post-operative complications, including a deformed appearance with the penis looking like it rises from the scrotum rather than the abdominal wall, and there is at least one report of a person dying from bleeding after penis augmentation.

Obese men appear to have a smaller penis because they develop a pad of fat in the pubic area and the flaccid penis becomes buried in it. So weight reduction is important before penis enlargement is considered. Very obese men might not be able to see their penis at all, because of their large and pendulous abdomen. Men should also remember that their penis will always look shorter when they look down at it, compared with looking straight at their penis in a mirror or across the changing room at another man's penis. This is a simple optical illusion.

Men who are born with a small penis may benefit from surgical treatment, but the results are unpredictable. Without surgery, many will still be able to enjoy very satisfactory sexual relationships despite the small size of their penis. Men who are dissatisfied with the appearance of their penis should think very carefully before requesting cosmetic surgery, especially if the size falls within the normal range. A better option may be to seek the advice of a sexual and relationship therapist, who might be able to offer help. The use of surgery to treat a psychological problem is fraught with risks. If surgery is the only way in which a man can regain his self-esteem and improve his self-image, he should seek advice from an experienced surgeon working in a reputable clinic.

UK cost (approx): Length and girth £6,200
See Section Two: Argentina

EAR RESHAPING

Bat ears, wing nuts, sticky-out-ears – call them what you like, they can be a source of both ridicule and teasing, especially for young children and teenagers. And they can lead youngsters to develop a complex about their looks that can have severe psychological consequences. The reason protruding ears are more noticeable in children is that by the age of four the ears are almost fully grown, so the earlier the surgery the less teasing the child will have to endure. But ear surgery, or otoplasty, is also possible on adults and there are no additional risks associated with an older patient.

About 2 per cent of people in the UK think their ears stick out too much, and the main treatment is an operation that reshapes the cartilage in the ear and uses plastic stitches to pin the ears back. In babies younger than about six months, it is possible to flatten the ears using special moulds to reshape the cartilage while it is still soft. Splints are fitted into the baby's ears, and left in place for weeks or months, depending on the age of the baby.

An otoplasty, also known as pinnaplasty, can be done under a general or local anaesthetic. The operation takes between one and two hours and is usually done as a day case with no overnight stay in hospital. With one of the more common techniques, the surgeon makes a small incision in the back of the ear to expose the ear cartilage. He or she will then sculpt the cartilage and bend it back towards the head. Non-removable stitches may be used to help maintain the new shape. Occasionally, the surgeon will remove a larger piece of cartilage to provide a more natural-looking fold when the surgery is complete. Another technique involves a similar incision in the back of the ear. Skin is removed and stitches are used to fold the cartilage back on itself to reshape the ear without removing cartilage. In most cases, ear surgery will leave a faint scar in the back of the ear that will fade with time. Even when only one ear appears to protrude, surgery is usually performed on both ears for a better balance.

Adults and children are usually up and around within a few hours of surgery. The patient's head will be wrapped in a bulky bandage immediately following surgery to promote the best moulding and healing. Once this large bandage has been removed, it may be necessary to wear a smaller and lighter headband for another few weeks – some people need to wear this day and night, others at nighttime only. The length of time the bandaging needs to be worn depends on the exact type of operation that is done. The surgeon will advise on when activities such as work or school can be resumed. It will not be possible to go swimming for at least two weeks, and contact sports should be avoided for around eight weeks.

Otoplasty is a commonly performed and generally safe surgical procedure, and for most people the benefits in terms of improved appearance are greater than any disadvantages.

UK cost (approx): £1,100–2,700
See Section Two: Argentina; Belgium; Czech
                   Republic; Germany; Hungary;
                   India; Mexico; Poland; South
                   Africa; Spain; Thailand; Tunisia;
                   Turkey

HAIR SURGERY

For something that we keep constantly cutting off as it grows, hair has a perverse hold over how human beings look and how we perceive ourselves. When hair stops growing and begins falling out, the first thing many people want to do is start putting it back.

Baldness is much more prevalent in men than women, is mainly hereditary and affects more than two-thirds of the male population. The hormone testosterone has a lot to do with it and explains why you may lose hair first from the front and top of the head but not the sides and back, which are not affected by hormones. You can also lose your hair because of an accident, disease or illness.

And there are plenty of old wives' tales about how to keep baldness at bay. If you get to 40 and show no signs of baldness, you never will; men who wear hats go bald quicker; vitamin deficiency, poor scalp circulation and even dandruff have been blamed. But keep your hair on – all these so-called theories have been disproved.

Anyone who elects for hair replacement must already have some hair on the back and sides of their head to act as donor areas. If you are completely bald, it is practically impossible to be treated. Replacement surgery can be quite a tricky procedure because there are many different transplant techniques involved, and most surgery involves combining quite a few techniques.

If you want just a modest change in the fullness of your hair, then a graft is probably the best way to go about it. There are slit grafts and strip grafts, micro- and mini-grafts and punch grafts. As the word implies, grafts are taken from an area of the head where there is hair and moved to an area of baldness. Grafts differ by size and shape. Round-shaped punch grafts usually contain about 10–15 hairs. The much smaller mini-graft contains about two to four hairs; and the micro-graft, one to two hairs. Slit grafts, which are inserted into slits created in the scalp, contain about four to 10 hairs each; strip grafts are long and thin and contain 30–40 hairs.

Although hair transplanting has improved enormously in recent years, it can still be a long process with many surgical sessions being needed with healing intervals of several months in between, and it can take up to two years before a final result is seen. But the results can be quite dramatic, as pop star Elton John will testify.

One step up from grafting is flap surgery, where a section of bald scalp is cut out and a flap of hair-bearing skin is lifted off the surface while still attached at one end. The hair-bearing flap is brought into its new position and sewn into place, while remaining 'tethered' to its original blood supply. One flap can be equal to more than 300 punch grafts.

Other techniques include scalp reduction, when hair-bearing scalp is pulled forward, and one that depends on a balloon-like device called a tissue-expander, which is inserted beneath the scalp and inflated with salt water over a period of weeks, causing the skin to expand and create new cells. Your surgeon will advise you on the best technique available depending on what kind of results you are expecting.

While hair surgery is usually a very safe technique there can be some risks, like excessive bleeding or wide scars known as 'stretch-back' scars. Many patients also find their 'new' hair falls out after about six weeks, but this is quite normal and it will grow again after another six weeks at around half an inch a month.

UK cost (approx): Micro-grafting £1,160–1,950 per session
See Section Two: Argentina; Czech Republic; Egypt; Italy; Poland; South Africa; Tunisia; Turkey

Chapter Three
DENTAL SURGERY

Nowadays, everybody, it seems, wants that 'Hollywood smile', the dazzling look that not merely brightens up the face but also adds a healthy appearance. But, as anyone who has ever been to Hollywood will know, dental surgery in America does not come cheap. Fortunately, dental practices all over the world are offering the same sort of treatment you would get in Hollywood, but for a fraction of the price.

The number of dental techniques and procedures available is quite staggering – and it would need a book much bigger than this guide to explain them all – but here are a few of the more frequent services. Always make sure you have a thorough consultation with your dental surgeon before any surgery begins, so that he or she knows exactly the finished effect you require.

ROOT CANAL TREATMENT
This is the treatment of the inner part of the tooth, known as the 'pulp tissue' but more popularly referred to as the

'nerve'. If the tooth's root degenerates then any inflammation can spread to the surrounding tissues. To prevent this happening, a dentist will remove any bacteria and organic debris from the inner aspects of the tooth and then fill in and seal off the interior of the tooth.

Root canal work is usually chosen because the teeth are one of the few places in the body where white blood cells can't reach to ward off infection, so abscesses can easily ensue. In a simplistic way, the dentist performs the job of the white blood cells by cleaning and sealing the area.

UK cost (approx): £300–700 per tooth
See Section Two: Argentina; Costa Rica; Croatia; Egypt; Hungary; India; Latvia; Mexico; South Africa; Thailand; Turkey

APICECTOMY

If an abscess has formed in the tooth root after it has already been filled, then the dentist will have to remove the tip of the root. It is usually done under local anaesthetic. A small cut is made to uncover the infected area, which is cleaned out with a small amount of surrounding bone removed. Sometimes new bone is grafted or the root filled and the gum stitched back into place. It takes about a week for the area to heal and you should rinse your mouth with a salt solution several times a day.

UK cost (approx): £250–300
See Section Two: Argentina; Costa Rica; Croatia;
                  Egypt; Hungary; India; Latvia;
                  South Africa; Thailand; Turkey

TEETH BLEACHING

There are different forms of teeth bleaching, from the whitening you can do at home to treatment by a professional dentist who uses an oxidising or bleaching agent to eliminate stains and discolouration caused by smoking, tea, coffee, wine or nerve degeneration. There is even whitening toothpaste although its effectiveness has not proved to be great.

The older method is for a dentist first to check that a patient has healthy and unrestored teeth, then take an impression of the upper and lower rows from which plaster moulds and trays are made to cover the teeth. These trays, which contain a bleaching solution, are worn for a couple of hours a day for up to six weeks.

A more popular modern method is to apply the bleaching solution straight on to the teeth and expose them to an intense light, which activates the bleach. The procedure takes only about 40 minutes, and then the teeth are polished.

Bleaching is successful in 90 per cent of patients and the effects can last for up to three years before another treatment is necessary. But side-effects can mean an increase in gum sensitivity, and bleaching doesn't lighten porcelain or silicates.

UK cost (approx): £300–1,300
See Section Two: Argentina; Costa Rica; Croatia;
                    Egypt; Hungary; India; Latvia;
                    Malaysia; Mexico; South Africa;
                    Thailand; Tunisia; Turkey

PORCELAIN TOOTH CROWNS

If your tooth has been affected by ageing, disease or breaking, then a crown can cover the entire visible surface of the tooth. The most aesthetically pleasing is the porcelain crown, although you can also have them in gold.

Crowns are usually made in a laboratory after the dentist has taken an impression of the tooth. The skill of the dentist is in fitting the crown and its colour, including the cement, so that it perfectly matches your other teeth. Crowns are very strong – much stronger than a filling – and a porcelain one is an excellent choice for front teeth.

UK cost (approx): £400–800 per crown
See Section Two: Argentina; Costa Rica; Croatia;
                    Egypt; Germany; Hungary; India;
                    Latvia; Malaysia; Mexico; Poland;
                    South Africa; Thailand; Tunisia;
                    Turkey

VENEERS

If you want great-looking teeth without all the hassle of crowns and braces, then the answer could be porcelain veneers. The veneer can hide a multitude of problems including gaps and badly aligned or out-of-shape teeth. It's as near as you can get to the instant answer for that 'Hollywood smile'. The dentist will tell you what it is possible to do with your teeth, and then he or she may do some minor contouring of the teeth and take an impression. The veneers are tried and, if suitable, bonded into place. The results can be spectacular.

But prices can rise quite steeply with veneers – even for the medical tourist – because you may need some new porcelain crowns as well, and you will end up with a complete makeover. There is very little downside in having teeth veneers. There is an adjustment period as the patient gets used to the size and shape of the 'new' teeth, and you must have realistic expectations. Although the veneers are reasonable facsimiles of natural teeth, they are not perfect replacements.

UK cost (approx): £300–500 per veneer
See Section Two: Argentina; Costa Rica; Croatia; Egypt; Germany; Hungary; India; Latvia; Malaysia; Poland; South Africa; Thailand; Turkey

IMPLANTS

In the old days, people would replace lost teeth with bridges or removable partial dentures, but now the more modern approach is with dental implants. These are fixtures of titanium that are specially screwed into the jawbone to hold a replacement tooth. Dentists maintain implants restore the proper chewing function, eliminate painful and irritated gums, stop progressive bone loss and support natural-looking teeth.

With root form implants, the dentist makes incisions in the gum down to the jawbone; the number of incisions depends on how many implants are to be placed. The implants are put in place and the gums stitched. Healing can take from three to six months while the bone grows in and around the implant, forming a strong support.

After the healing process is finished, the implant is uncovered and an 'abutment' attached to it. Now it's ready for your new tooth. For people with a narrow jawbone, another procedure called the plate implant is used. Once again, there is a healing period before the abutment and tooth can be attached. Since the implants are made of titanium, there is no chance of the body rejecting them.

UK cost (approx): £1,500–2,000 per tooth
See Section Two: Argentina; Costa Rica; Croatia;
                   Egypt; Germany; Hungary; India;
                   Latvia; Mexico; Poland; South
                   Africa; Thailand; Tunisia; Turkey

Chapter Four

EYE SURGERY

Think of the eye as if it is a camera. The cornea and lens are at the front like a camera lens; the retina, located at the back, is like the camera's film. In a normal eye, the image is focused perfectly on the retina. In nearsightedness, or myopia, the image is in front of – not on – the retina. This means that near images are clear but those far away are not. In farsightedness (hyperopia), the opposite happens. The light rays are not focused by the time they reach the retina and so near images are not clear while distant images are. Spectacles and contact lenses are able to correct these deficiencies, but more people are turning to surgery for a permanent solution.

With astigmatism, the rays of light form a line on the retina instead of a point and laser surgery is generally needed for its treatment. There is also presbyopia or 'ageing eye', which usually occurs in people between the ages of 40 and 50, and can be corrected with bifocals or reading glasses.

LASIK

LASIK eye surgery is the latest way of correcting vision problems. LASIK stands for 'Laser-Assisted In Situ Keratomileusis' and has advantages over other procedures because there is almost no pain and good vision is achieved immediately, or the next day at the latest. Basically, LASIK surgery changes the shape of the cornea permanently. A surgeon cuts a flap in the cornea, which is folded back to reveal the middle section of the cornea, called the stroma. A computer-controlled laser is used to vaporise a portion of the stroma and then the cornea flap is replaced.

Both near-sighted and far-sighted people can benefit from LASIK procedures by either flattening or steepening the cornea. Astigmatism can also be corrected by making the cornea a more normal shape.

Before deciding whether you need LASIK surgery, your ophthalmologist will make a thorough test of your eyes. As well as the usual tests, like using a slit lamp to look into the back of the eye and a tonometer to take the pressure of the eye, he or she will almost certainly use a corneal topographer, which creates a sort of 'map' of your cornea. From this 'map', the ophthalmologist can see any irregularities, and how steep or flat the cornea might be, and so judge what laser surgery is needed.

The surgery itself takes only a few minutes and you will be awake all the time, your eyes having been anaesthetised with special drops. Your eye will be positioned under the laser and held open by a suction ring retainer. A computer is used to make sure the laser is exactly adjusted for your prescription and then light pulses painlessly to remove stroma tissue.

After a rest, you should be able to go home and even back to work the next day, although as with all post-surgery it is advised that you take things easy to maximise healing and put no stress on the eyes.

If your cornea is too thin or too flat for LASIK surgery, there is a new technique called LASEK (Laser Epithelial Keratomileusis) in which the surgeon uses a much finer blade to cut the outer layer of the cornea and make the flap.

Bear in mind that LASIK and LASEK surgery treatments do not always work and a reduction in night vision is a very real possibility. It's not for everyone.

UK cost (approx): £1,000 per eye
See Section Two: Argentina; Belgium; Egypt;
                    India; Malaysia; South Africa;
                    Tunisia; Turkey

CATARACTS

The lens of the eye is enclosed in a capsule. As old cells die, they accumulate in the capsule, causing the lens to cloud over forming a cataract. This can take months or even years to happen and is the most common form of impaired vision in elderly people, who may see images as fuzzy or blurred. Cataract sufferers may also see haloes around lights. As well as the ageing process, diabetes or steroid abuse can cause the onset of cataracts. Smoking and drinking doesn't help either. If left untreated, cataracts may eventually cause blindness.

The most common method of cataract removal is for the eye to be numbed with an anaesthetic solution. The surgeon then makes an opening through the capsule and breaks up and removes the cloudy part of the lens using ultrasound or laser waves. An artificial lens is implanted at the same time that the cataract is removed. There may be swelling of the eye after the operation but infection is rare; the patient is usually given eye drops or antibiotic ointment and can resume normal activities the following day.

Glasses need to be worn after a cataract has been removed so that the light is focused on the retina, and if you already wear glasses then the prescription will need to be changed. The success rate of cataract removal is very high and affords sufferers a new lease of life.

UK cost (approx): £1,800–2,900
See Section Two: Argentina; Belgium; Cyprus;
                   France; Germany; India;
                   South Africa; Tunisia

Chapter Five

FERTILITY TREATMENT

It seems fertility treatment is never out of the newspapers. Only last year a Scottish woman aged 52 gave birth to twins after having fertility treatment abroad. She had been denied the treatment in Scotland because of her age.

But forget the sensationalist headlines, because infertility means heartbreak for thousands of ordinary couples who, try as hard as they might, are unable to have the family they so much desire. It can destroy marriages by tearing apart even the closest of partnerships.

Fortunately, in recent years, there have been advances in fertility treatment and since April 2005 women between the ages of 23 and 39 are able to get one free IVF cycle on the NHS. However, there are eligibility criteria and one cycle may not be enough. Private treatment can cost thousands of pounds, which is why more and more couples are looking abroad.

If considering fertility treatment, make sure you know

how fully experienced the doctor and his team are and the kind of laboratory being used. They can all add to your chances of achieving conception.

IN VITRO FERTILISATION

In vitro fertilisation (IVF) is the most common of the high-tech treatments and can help with ovulation problems, blocked fallopian tubes and low sperm count. At the beginning of a woman's menstrual cycle, she will be given a fertility drug, such as clomiphene, for the ovaries to develop mature eggs. Once mature, the eggs will be removed by needle through the vaginal wall – an anaesthetic is used – and combined in a laboratory with the partner's sperm. Two to four of the resulting embryos are then placed back in the uterus, while others may be frozen. If the treatment works, one of the embryos should grow into a baby.

Because of the wait for the eggs to mature, one cycle of IVF can take up to six weeks and there is about a 30 per cent chance of conceiving a child, depending on the age of the woman. The high cost involved with IVF is because of the expensive lab work required in fertilising an egg outside the body. The main complication is multiple births, which is directly attributed to putting multiple embryos into the uterus. If one of the embryos itself splits, which is rare, it would lead to an identical twin.

UK cost (approx): Two cycles £4,500+
See Section Two: Argentina; Belgium; Greece;
                   Hungary; India; Malaysia;
                   South Africa; Turkey

INTRA-CYTOPLASMIC SPERM INJECTION

In cases of severe male infertility, sperm are incapable of penetrating the outer layer of the egg and so IVF treatment is not recommended. The intra-cytoplasmic sperm injection (ICSI) technique assists penetration by injecting a single sperm directly into the egg. The treatment has been available since the early 1990s, and statistics show a high fertilisation rate with an overall pregnancy and live birth rate of above 30 per cent.

UK cost (approx): £3,780
See Section Two: Belgium; Greece; Hungary; India;
                   Malaysia; South Africa; Turkey

TESTICULAR SPERM ASPIRATION

Some men may have no sperm in their ejaculate for different reasons, such as a failed vasectomy reversal or a previous severe infection. Or they may be unable to ejaculate due to spinal cord injuries.

With testicular sperm aspiration (TESA), sperm is harvested directly from the testes by putting a needle into the testicle while the patient is under local anaesthetic. The sperm can be used in IVF or ICSI treatment and, once fertilised, the embryo is implanted into the uterus.

UK cost (approx): £1,320
See Section Two: Belgium; India; Malaysia;
                   South Africa; Hungary; Turkey

Chapter Six

GENDER REASSIGNMENT

Gender-reassignment therapy is an umbrella term for all medical procedures regarding gender reassignment of both transgendered and intersexual people. It is sometimes called a sex change and consists of hormone replacement therapy (HRT), various surgical procedures, and epilation for transwomen – permanent hair removal on the face and body accomplished with electrolysis or laser hair removal.

The requirements for HRT vary greatly. Often, at least a certain amount of psychological counselling is required, and so also is a time of living in the desired gender role, if possible, to ensure that the patient can psychologically function in that life-role. This period is sometimes called the Real Life Test (RLT).

Generally speaking, physicians who perform sex-reassignment surgery require the patient to live as the opposite gender in all possible ways ('cross-live') for at least a year prior to the start of surgery. The RLT is usually part of a battery of requirements. Other frequent requirements are regular psychological counselling and letters of recommendation for gender-reassignment surgery.

TRANSMEN (direction female–to–male)

Many transmen do not opt for genital-reassignment surgery, but almost all undergo a double mastectomy and the shaping of a masculine chest, a hysterectomy and the removal of internal female sex organs, along with hormone treatment with testosterone.

MASTECTOMY

Most transmen require bilateral mastectomy – the removal of female breasts and the shaping of a male-contoured chest. Transmen with moderate to large breasts usually require a formal bilateral mastectomy with grafting and reconstruction of the nipple-areola. This will result in two horizontal scars on the lower edge of the pectoral muscle, but allows for easier resizing of the nipple and placement in a typically male position.

Some doctors perform the surgery in two steps: first, the contents of the breast are removed through a cut either inside or around the areola, and the skin is allowed to retract for about a year; then, in a second surgical procedure, the excess skin is removed. This technique results in far less scarring than the next procedure, and the nipple-areola doesn't need to be removed and grafted.

Complete removal of the breast and grafting often results in a loss of sensation of that area that may take from six months to over a year to return, or it may never return at all, and in rare cases results in the complete loss of sensation in this tissue. In these uncommon situations, a nipple can be reconstructed as it is for women whose nipples are removed as part of treatment for breast cancer.

For transmen with smaller breasts, a peri-areolar or 'keyhole' procedure may be done where the mastectomy is performed through an incision made around the areola. This avoids the larger scars of a traditional mastectomy, but the nipples may be larger and may not be in a perfectly male orientation on the chest wall. In addition, there is less denervation (damage to the nerves supplying the skin) of the chest wall with a peri-areolar mastectomy, and less time is required for sensation to return.

HYSTERECTOMY AND BILATERAL SALPINGO-OOPHORECTOMY

Hysterectomy is the removal of the uterus. Bilateral salpingo-oophorectomy (BSO) is the removal of both ovaries and fallopian tubes. Hysterectomy without BSO in cisgendered (not transgendered) women is sometimes referred to as a 'partial hysterectomy', and is done to treat uterine disease while maintaining the female hormonal milieu until natural menopause occurs.

Some transmen desire to have a hysterectomy/BSO because of a discomfort with having internal female reproductive organs, despite the fact that menses usually cease with hormonal therapy. Some undergo this as their only gender-identity-confirming 'bottom surgery'.

For many transmen, however, hysterectomy/BSO is done to decrease the risk of developing cervical, endometrial and ovarian cancer (although, like breast cancer, the risk does not become zero but is drastically decreased). Whether gynaecologic cancers are increased in transmen is not known, and unfortunately will never be known. This is for the same reason that assaying the risk of rare diseases in small populations is often impossible. The numbers are too small to make a valid epidemiological conclusion even if every member of the population were involved in a study.

Decreasing cancer risk is particularly important, however, as transmen often feel uncomfortable seeking gynaecologic care, and many do not have access to adequate and culturally sensitive treatment. Ideally, though, even after hysterectomy/BSO, transmen should see a gynaecologist for a check-up at least every three years. This is particularly the case for transmen who retain their vagina (whether before or after further genital reconstruction); have a strong family history of cancers of the breast, ovary or uterus (endometrium); have a personal history of gynaecological cancer or significant dysplasia on a cervical smear.

One important consideration for any transman who develops vaginal bleeding after successfully ceasing menses on testosterone is that he must be evaluated by a gynaecologist. This is equivalent to post-menopausal bleeding in a cisgendered woman and may herald the development of a gynaecologic cancer.

GENITAL REASSIGNMENT

Genital-reconstructive procedures (GRT) use either the clitoris, which is enlarged by androgenic hormones, or rely on free tissue grafts from the arm, thigh or belly and an erectile prosthesis. The latter usually include multiple procedures, more expense and have a less satisfactory outcome, in terms of replicating nature.

In either case, the urethra can be rerouted through the phallus to allow urination through the reconstructed penis. The labia major are united to form a scrotum, where prosthetic testicles can be inserted.

TRANSWOMEN (direction male–to–female)

Sex-reassignment surgery from male to female includes surgeries that will shape a male body into a body with the appearance and, as far as possible, the functioning of a female body.

Christine Jorgensen is likely to have been the most famous recipient of sex-reassignment surgery, having had her surgery done in Denmark in late 1952 and being outed right afterwards by the *New York Daily News*. She was a strong advocate for the rights of transsexual people, touring until her death in 1989. Another famous person to undergo male-to-female sex-reassignment surgery was Dr Renee Richards. She transitioned and had surgery in the mid-1970s, and successfully fought to have transsexual people recognised in their new sex. She herself played professional tennis.

GENITAL–REASSIGNMENT SURGERY

Primary male-to-female (MTF) procedures fall under one of two categories: penile inversion or (less commonly) colovaginoplasty. Sex-reassignment surgery (SRS) can be completed in either a single surgery or two surgeries, depending on the surgeon's technique.

For changing anatomical sex from male to female, the testicles are removed and the penis is usually inverted to form a vagina (vaginoplasty) or, if additional depth or self-lubrication is desired, a section of colon may be grafted in (colovaginoplasty). For additional vaginal depth, pubic hairs are removed from scrotal tissues via electrolysis prior to the SRS procedure. The tissues are then incorporated by the surgeon to extend the vaginal shaft, where penile tissues alone were found to be insufficient. If either technique performed involves two surgeries, the second surgery is a minor surgery called labiaplasty.

A third, crudest form of reassignment is where the penile tissue is removed altogether (penectomy) and vaginal tissue created from grafts.

Any technique of vaginoplasty performed will require vaginal dilation of the patient for the rest of her life with a set of vaginal stents. This is due to the body treating the vagina as a wound, thus trying to close it. Dilation is started several days after surgery, when the temporary packing inserted during surgery is removed. After several weeks of several dilations per day, the patients will eventually be able to cut down to one dilation per week. It is important to note that sexual intercourse does not count as a dilation; the body requires the hard presence of the stents to keep the vagina from losing depth.

BREAST AUGMENTATION

Breast augmentation is the enlargement of breasts, which can be necessary if hormone therapy did not yield satisfactory results. (See Cosmetic Surgery)

FACIAL-FEMINISATION SURGERY

Occasionally, these basic procedures are complemented further with feminising cosmetic surgeries or procedures that modify bone or cartilage structures, typically in the jaw, brow, forehead, nose and cheek areas. (See Cosmetic Surgery)

VOICE SURGERY

Some MTF individuals may elect to have voice surgery to alter the range or pitch of their vocal cords. Oestrogens by themselves are not able to alter the voice range or pitch. Voice lessons are available to train the MTF to practise feminisation of their speech.

TRACHEAL SHAVES

Tracheal shaves are available to reduce the cartilage in

the area of the throat to conform to more feminine dimensions.

(This article is licensed under GNU Free Documentation Licence. It uses material from the Wikipedia article Gender Reassignment Therapy – http://en.wikipedia.org/wiki/Gender_reassignment_therapy.)

UK cost (approx): £30,000+
See Section Two: Thailand

Chapter Seven

GENERAL SURGERY

CARPAL TUNNEL SYNDROME

Carpal tunnel syndrome occurs when the nerve running from the forearm to the hand becomes squeezed at the wrist resulting in pain, weakness or numbness in the hand. Symptoms start gradually with tingling or burning, most notably at night, and eventually lead to decreased grip strength and the sufferer continually having to shake out their hand. Women are three times more likely than men to develop the syndrome and it can be caused by everything from repetitive strain to genetic inheritance.

Non-surgical treatments include anti-inflammatory drugs like Ibuprofen, exercise and acupuncture, but if symptoms last for more than six months then surgery may be required.

The surgery is fairly simple. Local anaesthetic is injected into the wrist or higher up the arm, then the ligament that forms the roof of the carpal tunnel is cut and the pressure on the nerve is released. It can be done as an outpatient procedure and patients are generally not required to stay overnight.

Tingling may continue to occur in the hand for some time and dressings should be left on for five days. After surgery, it is rare for carpal tunnel syndrome to return, although it is not unknown.

UK cost (approx): £700–1,600
See Section Two: Belgium; Hungary; India;
                    South Africa

GALLBLADDER REMOVAL/CHOLECYSTECTOMY

The gallbladder is an organ positioned next to the liver from which it collects bile. It sends the bile to the small intestine through ducts and the bile aids digestion. The gall bladder is not a vital organ and the body can cope quite well without it. If the excess cholesterol in the bile crystallises, it can form gallstones; these can lead to pain and complications such as jaundice, gall-bladder infections, inflammation of the pancreas and very rarely cancer of the gallbladder. If many gallstones are detected in a person's gallbladder, then they may be advised to have the gallbladder removed altogether. This can be done by laparoscopic (keyhole) surgery, as well as the more traditional open surgery. In both cases, the operation is similar.

With the laparoscopic approach, the surgeon makes a number of small incisions in the abdomen and, using a minute camera attached to the laparoscope, examines the gallbladder. He or she clips shut the ducts and arteries that service the bladder and then cuts it free, removing it along with its gallstones back through one of the small incisions.

With open surgery, the hospital stay can be up to eight days; with laparoscopic, it can be one or two days. After surgery, you should rest for up to five days and avoid any heavy lifting. You should expect the digestive system to take a few days to settle down, which means you may feel bloated and have a change of toilet habits.

UK cost (approx): £3,500–5,800
See Section Two: Belgium; Hungary; India; Malaysia; South Africa

GALLSTONE REMOVAL/CHOLELITHOTOMY

When gallstones form due to the crystallisation of aggregate in the gallbladder, they move around the bladder and block the ducts, preventing the bladder from emptying its bile. This can result in inflammation, irritation and infection of the gallbladder. Overweight middle-aged women are the most prone to gallstones.

The stones can cause serious trouble if, for instance, one of them has travelled down the cystic duct or bile ducts and become stuck there. They can lead to pancreatitis, as well as cause severe attacks of pain in the upper abdomen.

Most gallstones are extracted by the complete

removal of the gallbladder (see above) – this is the procedure of choice in most patients because once the bladder is removed the stones will not reoccur.

But there are other treatments, especially for people deemed too old or frail to undergo surgery. In the case of stones caused purely by cholesterol, methods may be used to dissolve them. A catheter is inserted into the gallbladder and a small amount of solvent is continuously pumped in, but this is neither simple nor particularly safe.

Another method is to destroy the stones by bombarding them with ultrasonic waves, but this can only be done for small stones and the success rate is little better than 50/50. For the best type of treatment, seek medical advice.

UK cost (approx): See gallbladder removal
See Section Two: Belgium; Hungary; India;
                   South Africa

GASTRIC BYPASS AND LAP BAND

A gastric bypass is an extreme operation elected by patients who are morbidly obese, and seemingly can't do anything about it. Its results are startling, though, and for many people whose life may be threatened by their incredible weight it is literally a lifeline. As people in the western world, especially the USA and UK, become more obese, gastric bypasses are increasing in popularity. Many surgeons will not even consider patients for a gastric bypass unless they are at least 100lbs overweight and have exhausted every other avenue of losing weight, including strict dieting and exercise. The simple reason is that it is not a quick fix – it's major surgery, sometimes known as stomach stapling, and requires the patient to commit him- or herself to a lifetime of eating well and staying fit. The idea is to make the stomach smaller and let food bypass part of the small intestine. The result is that you feel full more quickly and so reduce the amount of food you eat.

There are two procedures: an open procedure, which involves making a large incision; and another newer procedure using small incisions and involving microsurgery with the use of a camera, known as a laparoscopic approach. In both procedures, a pouch is created at the top of the stomach using staples or a plastic band. The pouch is then connected to the middle portion of the small intestine, bypassing the rest of the stomach. It means the stomach is now just a small pouch. The beauty of the lap band, unlike staples, is that it is fully reversible simply by removing the band.

The results can be quite spectacular with patients losing weight quickly and continuing to lose weight for up to 12 months. But staying healthy is an ongoing process because the part of the intestine that is bypassed is the part where minerals and vitamins are most easily absorbed, so nutrient supplements are advised as well as the help of a dietician to prevent long-term problems of deficiency in iron, calcium or vitamins.

You will usually need to stay in hospital for four to five days after gastric-bypass surgery and will remain on liquid or puréed food for several weeks until you can start on small bits of solids. You can generally resume exercise six weeks after the operation. Even sooner than that, you will be able to take short walks at a comfortable pace.

UK cost (approx): £6,500–8,000
See Section Two: Belgium; Germany; Hungary; India; Malaysia; South Africa

HAEMORRHOIDECTOMY

Haemorrhoids or 'piles' have always been sniggered at as if they were a bit of a joke, but they are no joke if you suffer from them. We all have haemorrhoids inside the anus and they are useful things because they help us to stop passing wind and motions until we are ready. But because they contain many blood vessels they bleed easily, and something like 20 per cent of the UK population have problems with haemorrhoids. A high-fibre diet is advised to keep the haemorrhoids in good condition.

Small problem haemorrhoids can be treated at an outpatients' clinic, but larger ones may require an operation. The operation is fairly simple. You are given a general anaesthetic, the ring muscle is stretched and, either by using a freezing technique or rubber bands, the piles are cut off.

After the operation, there is a little discomfort when moving and the bowels may not open for a day or so. But once this happens you will be able to leave hospital and by the end of the first week you should be pain-free.

Complications are rare and seldom serious. The operation has a reputation for being painful but in fact is less troublesome than people are led to believe, although it may be a month before things are back to normal.

UK cost (approx): £1,400–2,750
See Section Two: Belgium; Hungary; India; Poland; South Africa

ABDOMINAL HERNIA

Everyone, from newborn babies to old-age pensioners, can develop an abdominal hernia, which is when part of the intestines protrudes through the abdominal wall. It is given different names depending on the area in which it occurs, but is noticeable as a bulge that may appear bigger when standing up and smaller when lying down.

Most hernias are caused by a weakness in the abdominal wall, which can be exacerbated by factors like heavy lifting, pregnancy, straining and obesity. Some hernias can be reduced by a doctor simply pushing the bulge back into place. But, once an abdominal hernia occurs, it tends to increase in size; surgical treatment may be the only answer, because if the intestines become trapped outside the abdomen it could lead to a cut off in blood supply, known as a 'strangulated hernia'.

Surgical repair is not as difficult as one might think. It involves making an abdominal incision either conventionally or with a laparoscope (keyhole surgery), and the surgeon either pushing the protruding tissue back into the abdomen or removing it. The area can be stitched up or, if it is particularly weak, strengthened with either a special type of mesh or the surrounding muscle.

Recovery can be quite quick depending on where the hernia is, but in all cases it is necessary to rest and avoid any heavy lifting during recuperation. The patient can expect total recovery in two to four weeks.

UK cost (approx): £1,300–2,450
See Section Two: Belgium; Hungary; India; Malaysia; Poland; South Africa

HYDROCELE

The main symptom of a hydrocele is a painless but swollen testicle – it can be one or both – which feels like a water-filled balloon.

Hydroceles are quite common in newborn babies and, while they may worry the parents, they usually resolve themselves after a few months. It is a hydrocele in an older man, caused by inflammation or trauma of the testicle, which often needs attention. The fluid in the hydrocele is usually clear and a doctor can shine a light through the scrotum to outline the testicle and indicate the presence of the fluid.

Hydroceles are not particularly dangerous but they can cause embarrassment and discomfort. The simplest method of treatment is to aspirate the scrotum, which means putting a needle into the hydrocele and withdrawing the fluid. However, hydroceles can reoccur after an aspiration.

The alternative is an operation under general anaesthetic in which a small incision is made in the scrotum and the hydrocele sac removed. The scrotum is then repaired with dissolving stitches. In either case, swelling of the scrotum following an operation is common, and the patient should rest for a week, wearing an athletic support.

Hydroceles can be left untreated but they may get bigger, so it is best to have any enlargement of the testicles checked out.

UK cost (approx): £1,700–2,300
See Section Two: Belgium; Hungary; India; Malaysia; South Africa

HYSTERECTOMY

A hysterectomy is a removal of the uterus (womb) and there may be many reasons why a woman might want or need to have it done. Cancer of the uterus almost always means a hysterectomy is necessary, but some women elect to have the procedure because it will improve the quality of their life if they suffer from heavy bleeding, chronic pain or discomfort. A qualified doctor should decide whether a patient's condition merits a hysterectomy. Although it is a major operation, the surgical risks are low. However, only women who do not wish to have children in the future should opt for such a procedure.

Hysterectomies can be done through the vagina, which leaves no external signs, with keyhole surgery, or through the abdomen. The latter is the most common procedure, leaving a six-inch scar across the lower abdomen known as a bikini cut because it runs across the top of the pubic hairline. This form of operation allows the surgeon to see the pelvic area, giving him a bigger operating space, but it means patients stay in hospital longer than if it was a vaginal hysterectomy.

Complete recovery takes about six to eight weeks and the hospital stay can last for between three and seven days. After the operation, the patient will no longer have menstrual periods and no longer be able to get pregnant, but it usually has no effect on the ability to experience sexual pleasure and orgasm. In fact, many women find the sexual experience more enjoyable because there is no longer any fear of becoming pregnant.

UK cost (approx):   £4,000–5,050
See Section Two: Belgium; Hungary; India; Malaysia;
                   South Africa

PROSTATE REMOVAL

The prostate is a gland found only in men, under the bladder and in front of the rectum, and is the size of a walnut. It creates a fluid that makes up 15 per cent of male semen and helps to sustain sperm cells. The prostate is surrounded by muscle, which contracts during ejaculation. Its removal may be recommended when a patient is diagnosed with prostate cancer or the prostate has become greatly enlarged.

The type of surgery used depends on the size of the prostate. The most common is transurethral, also known as a TURP procedure, in which a tube-like instrument is inserted into the penis and the gland is cut away piece by piece. It is fine for small prostates and doesn't leave an external incision. If the surgeon judges the prostate to be bigger than 80 grams, then open surgery is used, with an incision made between the belly-button and the penis. This procedure requires a longer stay in hospital and longer recovery. Newer treatments include laser incisions, microwave therapy and balloon dilation of the urethra.

The stay in hospital can last for around seven days and complete recovery takes about three weeks. Apart from the usual risks associated with any major surgery, such as anaesthetic reaction or infection, some patients may have problems with urine control and achieving and maintaining an erection.

UK cost (approx): £3,650–4,650
See Section Two: Belgium; Cyprus; France; Germany;
                    Hungary; India;
                    South Africa

WRIST TENDONITIS

When the tendons around the wrist joint become inflamed, the area can be very painful with swelling of the surrounding soft tissues, and a doctor might suggest a few different courses of treatment. The wrist can be put in a splint and rested with an ice pack to help the swelling go down. Anti-inflammatory medicines might be used, and even cortisone injected right into the site of the inflammation.

If none of these approaches works, surgery is the solution. In such cases, the surgeon makes an incision to release the area of tight tendon, and inflammatory tissue may be removed to allow the tendon to move more freely.

UK cost (approx): £700–1,600
See Section Two: Belgium; Hungary; India;
                    South Africa

TONSILLECTOMY

Your tonsils are the two lumps of tissue found on each side of the back of your throat. They can become infected – especially in children. If antibiotics fail to stop recurring tonsillitis then your doctor may suggest that they be removed. It is one of the most common surgical procedures in the world and requires merely a day in hospital.

Under general anaesthetic, the surgeon simply cuts out the tonsil tissue and cauterises the area to control bleeding. There may be a little discomfort after the operation, ironically similar to the pain of tonsillitis, but this will be controlled with pain medication. Recovery is very quick.

While general surgery is still the most common procedure for people suffering from tonsillitis, newer treatments are also becoming available. These include cold ablation and the use of lasers and ultrasound.

UK cost (approx): £1,550–2,150
See Section Two: Belgium; Hungary; India;
                   South Africa

Chapter Eight

ORTHOPAEDIC SURGERY

Orthopaedic operations, alongside cosmetic surgery and dental treatment, are the most popular procedures for medical tourists. The cost of orthopaedic operations abroad can often be half what you would pay privately in the UK, and in the case of India only a quarter as much.

The word orthopaedic is from the Greek for 'straight child', and started off literally as limb and spine straightening. Modern techniques have now made orthopaedic procedures some of the most successful medical operations available.

TOTAL HIP REPLACEMENT

The hip is simply a sophisticated ball-and-socket joint with the head of the thighbone (femur) as the ball and the pelvic cup (acetabulum) as the socket. Strong ligaments hold the ball in the socket, both of which are covered with a smooth layer of soft white substance known as cartilage, which allows for easy movement and no friction.

The wear and tear of the ageing process can slowly damage and destroy the cartilage until there is nothing left of the soft cushion. This is known as osteoarthritis and can be painful and disabling. Osteoarthritis can also be brought on in people who are overweight or if the joint has been damaged by injury or a fall. In many cases, osteoarthritis demands a hip replacement for the patient to be fully mobile again, although painkillers, use of a walking stick, weight loss and physiotherapy can help to lessen the pain.

During surgery, the head of the femur is cut off and replaced with a new ball attached to a metal implant inside the femur bone. Damaged cartilage and bone is removed from the hip socket using a reaming device, and a metal shell put inside the socket. Traditionally, the new ball has been made of metal and the new socket shell lined with polyethylene, and this is still the preferred method for elderly patients. But advances in medicine have seen people being given metal-to-metal replacements, which last longer than metal-to-polyethylene and, more recently, ceramic-to-ceramic, which has very low friction, may last for up to 40 years and is ideal for younger patients.

The metal implant inside the femur, which holds the ball in place, may be either pressed in place, or in some cases cemented. The total time for the operation is around two to three hours.

Conventional hip-replacement surgery usually requires an incision of eight to twelve inches. The latest minimally invasive technique, however, uses two much smaller incisions whereby the surgeon operates between muscles, tendons and ligaments rather than cutting through them. Proponents of the new technique maintain patients leave hospital and walk sooner, and can resume everyday activities much more quickly.

Your stay in hospital will be between five and ten days, you will leave walking with sticks or crutches and you will not be able to drive for up to six weeks. Preparation for the operation and aftercare is as important as the procedure itself.

As with any surgery, there are risks with a total hip replacement (THR) procedure, including post-operative deep vein thrombosis, dislocation – when the ball comes out of the socket – and unequal leg lengths. But 90 per cent of patients have no problems whatsoever and a THR is one of the most successful operations you can have.

UK cost (approx): £7,000–8,900
See Section Two: Belgium; Cyprus; France; Germany; Hungary; India; Malaysia; Poland; South Africa; Thailand

REVISION HIP REPLACEMENT
With an older-style metal-to-polyethylene total hip replacement, eventually the polyethylene will start to

wear away through friction. When this may happen is unknown. Some replacements last longer than others, but a day may come when a patient needs a 'revision'. It is less common if newer materials, like metal-to-metal or ceramic-to-ceramic, have been used in the initial operation. It's not just wear that can lead to a revision. Bone loss, joint loosening, fracture, dislocation and infection can also lead to the need for a new operation.

Revision surgery is more complicated and takes longer than the original operation, not only because the patient is now older; it also depends on the quality of the bone and the ability to secure the replacement elements into position.

Before thinking about a revision, patients must talk through all alternative possibilities with their doctor, because revision surgery is one of the most difficult of orthopaedic procedures. A mini-incision operation is not possible as it is with a THR, and much depends on how difficult it is to remove the metal prosthesis inside the femur. Wires and bone grafts may also be needed, which can lead to a higher incidence of infection.

UK cost (approx): £11,500–13,000
See Section Two: Belgium; France; Hungary; India;
                 Malaysia; Poland; South Africa;
                 Thailand

HIP RESURFACING

Whereas a THR operation replaces both the socket and

ball, a resurface merely replaces the socket and puts a new surface on the femoral head instead of replacing the ball. This means there is very little bone removed and no need for a large metal prosthesis to be implanted in the femur. If revision surgery is ever needed, it means there will be more bone for the surgeon to play with.

The procedure, which uses metal-to-metal, is usually offered to younger patients (under the age of 55) who want to maintain an active lifestyle. Resurfacing creates a bigger ball, which makes dislocation less likely, and the whole operation can be done in 90 minutes instead of up to three hours.

The procedure is often called the 'Birmingham hip' after the two doctors in Birmingham, England, who developed the technique, and has been used worldwide for more than 10 years. It is a technically demanding operation, more so than a THR, although the basics of the operation are similar (see above). The main disadvantage is the fact that no one knows the long-term effects of the procedure and there is a small risk of the femur fracturing during or after surgery.

In most cases, patients are back to work within three months, free of a walking stick or crutches and sleeping on the operated side.

UK cost (approx): £10,000–12,500
See Section Two: Belgium; France; Hungary; India;
                  Malaysia; South Africa; Thailand

KNEE REPLACEMENT

As the population grows older, artificial knee replacements are becoming more popular. Once again, osteoarthritis, due to the wearing away of the cartilage inside the joint, is to blame. Fractures of the knee, torn cartilages and torn ligaments can also hasten the onset of osteoarthritis. Pain can be considerable and the sufferer may not be able to straighten the knee, which can become swollen with fluid. As with degenerative hips, the first course of action may be painkillers and a walking stick.

An operation, also known as a total knee arthroplasty, involves the surgeon exposing the capsule surrounding the knee joint, opening it and removing the ends of the thighbone (femur), shinbone (tibia) and often the underside of the kneecap (patella). A metal shell is put on the end of the femur, a metal and plastic trough on the tibia and, if needed, a plastic button on the kneecap. The artificial parts are cemented into place and the procedure may take between two and four hours.

Reports suggest that an artificial knee should last at least 10 years before it starts to 'loosen' because of activity or bone pulling away from the cement.

The operation is performed under general anaesthetic and once again the main post-operative risks, as with hip surgery, involve the danger of deep vein thrombosis and infection. As with hip replacement, rehabilitation and good after care is paramount.

The recovery time is about three months, with a week

or more spent in hospital, and total recovery – back to normal activities – can be up to a year, with low-impact activities like swimming and golf perfectly possible.

UK cost (approx): £8,800–10,300
See Section Two: Belgium; Cyprus; France; Germany;
                    Hungary; India; Malaysia; Poland;
                    South Africa; Thailand

REVISION KNEE REPLACEMENT

After 10 to 15 years, a total knee replacement may need revising and this is complex surgery that can mean up to three weeks in hospital. The problem here, if the replacement has 'loosened', is the removal of the prosthesis and the quality of bone left behind after it has been removed. A patient may require bone grafts from a bone bank.

Once the original prosthesis and cement have been removed and bone renovated, the revision surgery is similar to the original operation. However, the success rate is lower and complications can include easier dislocation and one leg becoming shorter than the other. Antibiotic cement may have to be used, followed by a course of antibiotics to prevent infection.

Knee revision surgery is more difficult than hip revision, and patients are asked to think carefully about whether or not their pain is manageable before electing to have the procedure.

UK cost (approx): £12,500–14,300
See Section Two: Belgium; Hungary; India; Malaysia;
Poland; South Africa; Thailand

KNEE ARTHROSCOPY

One of the most frequent procedures for the diagnosis and treatment of knee injuries is a knee arthroscopy. A small telescopic instrument with a lens and surgical attachments is inserted into the knee through small, minimally invasive incisions. The keyhole surgery allows surgeons to take tissue samples of the knee and also repair damage to cartilage.

The stay in hospital is short and sometimes not even overnight, while the arthroscopy takes between 30 minutes and an hour under general anaesthetic. After the operation, the patient may need to take painkillers for the soreness and the knee may feel stiff, but crutches are rarely needed.

UK cost (approx): £1,500–2,850
See Section Two: Belgium; Hungary; India; Malaysia;
Poland; South Africa; Thailand

OXFORD KNEE REPLACEMENT

The Oxford knee, also known as unicompartmental knee replacement, replaces just one side of the knee joint, unlike total knee replacement, which involves the removal of all surfaces of the joint. It is quite a technical feat to reconstruct one half of the joint while keeping the other half intact, especially as it is now usually performed with miniaturised instruments through an incision three inches long.

On the positive side, recovery takes only a third as long as a total replacement if keyhole surgery has been used, and there is much less pain. On the negative side, this seemingly revolutionary technique is not suitable for people suffering from rheumatoid arthritis or those where osteoarthritis has progressed too far and damaged the cruciate ligaments.

UK cost (approx): £9,000–11,500
See Section Two: Belgium; Hungary; India;
                   South Africa; Thailand

SHOULDER REPLACEMENT

The shoulder joint is a ball-and-socket joint much like the hip. This time the ball is the top of the arm-bone (humerus) and the socket is within the shoulder blade (scapula). The top of the arm-bone is coated with cartilage and an inner lining in the socket allows for smooth movement. Tendons and muscles give the joint support.

Once again, arthritis or degenerative disease can make the shoulder stiff and painful, and the ultimate answer can be to have replacement surgery with the damaged areas replaced with a prosthesis. Under general anaesthetic, the surgeon makes an incision of four to six inches from the collarbone to the upper arm-bone, which is then dislocated from the socket to expose the ball-like end of the humerus. It is cleaned and hollowed out to match the implant stem, and a correct-sized ball attached. Damaged cartilage is removed from the socket and it is then usually fitted with a polyethylene component, which is cemented into position. The arm-bone is replaced in the socket and the supporting tendons reattached.

The operation can take up to three hours and the hospital stay varies from one to three days. Patients will have to wear a sling and do strengthening exercises for the muscles around the shoulder. Within three months, they should be able to return to most normal activities, but must be aware of the risks of dislocation.

As with all orthopaedic replacement surgery, loosening can occur over time and a revision may be necessary years down the line.

UK cost (approx): £11,500–13,900
See Section Two: Belgium; Hungary; India; Malaysia; Poland; South Africa; Thailand

Chapter Nine
SCANS AND HEALTH CHECKS

Prevention, we are always told, is better than cure. And one of the best things anyone can do when they reach middle age is to have a full personal MOT. But, while we might be aware that a total health check is good for us, many people put it off because of cost. It's the 'I feel all right so why should I waste good money on having it proved to me?' attitude. Other people would rather not know if there are any impending problems and prefer to face them when they happen.

But health checks can be so much more affordable outside the UK that the wise tourist is taking a day – or half a day – out of his holiday to get checked out and scanned.

CT SCAN

A CT, or computed tomography, scan is sometimes known as a CAT scan and uses X-rays to get data from different angles around the body. This is then computer-processed and interpreted by radiologists to diagnose problems like heart disease, cancers and muscle disorders.

The patient is put on a CT table, which moves slowly into the scanner with its position depending on the area of the body to be examined. It causes no pain, although a contrast material like barium or water-soluble iodine may be swallowed or injected into the bloodstream to increase the visibility of certain blood vessels or tissues. One drawback is that it shows pictures only horizontally, but the examination is fast, simple, painless and accurate with the only risk really in being exposed to radiation, as one would be when having an X-ray.

Most scans take about half an hour and are quicker than an MRI scan. Having to lie still can be uncomfortable, though, and you have to remember not to cough or swallow, especially when the head is being scanned.

UK cost (approx): body scan £650; heart scan £350; lung scan £350; colon scan £500

See Section Two: Belgium; Costa Rica; India; Malaysia; Poland; South Africa

MRI SCAN

An MRI, or magnetic resonance imaging, scan has the advantage that there is no exposure to X-rays or radiation because it uses magnetic and radio waves. The actual scanner is a tube surrounded by a giant magnet. The magnet field aligns the hydrogen atoms and protons, which are then exposed to radio waves. The signal given off is processed by a computer, which produces an image.

In this way, it's possible to take pictures of almost all body tissue. Tissue with few hydrogen atoms, such as bone, appears dark, while that with lots of hydrogen atoms, like fatty tissue, looks brighter.

The MRI scan can create very detailed pictures and it is an excellent technique for diagnosing tumours in the brain. It's also good for scanning the heart and checking any defects that may have been building over time. MRI scans are often much clearer than CT scans and there are no known side-effects. It is also a totally painless procedure. The only real drawback is that people with any metal implants in their body, like pins or rods in their bones or a heart pacemaker, are not suitable for a scan because the magnet field attracts metal objects. For the same reason, metal objects like coins, jewellery, watches, piercings and even dentures must be removed before scanning.

The scan can be quite noisy, making a sort of clanging sound, and some patients are offered earplugs. The scan can take between 30 and 90 minutes and it can be a little uncomfortable staying still for that period of time.

UK cost (approx): single area £395; additional areas £195
See Section Two: Belgium; Costa Rica; India; Malaysia; Poland; South Africa; Thailand

PET SCAN

A PET, or positron emission tomography, scan is a nuclear medicine technique using a camera that captures powerful images of the body, showing its internal chemistry. It means that, unlike a CT or MRI scan, it can actually detect early chemical and metabolic changes in diseased states, making it ideal for the early diagnosis of cancers.

Patients are injected with a radioactive substance, which takes about half an hour to travel round the body and into the tissue to be examined. The actual scanning takes about 30 to 45 minutes. The patient's exposure to radiation is very low and of no danger, but pregnant women should inform the PET staff before the scanning takes place.

Sometimes PET scans are combined with an MRI or CT scan to get a full picture of a patient's health.

UK cost (approx): £800–1,000
See Section Two: Belgium; Costa Rica; India;
                   Malaysia; Poland; South Africa

HEALTH CHECKS

Having a total health check may seem a bit paranoid, especially if you appear to be in good health – and the price of a private hospital health check in the UK can be prohibitive. But in India, for instance, that check, which can detect any problems early on and point you towards a healthier lifestyle, can be only a tenth of the cost. It is something that can be done quickly in a day, and is worth bearing in mind while you are on your holiday.

Ideally, the following should be included in the ultimate health check, although it is not necessary that every test should be done:

Height/Weight/Body-fat tumour markers	Haematological parameters (AFP/CEA)
Gout	Diabetes mellitus
Urinalysis	Audiometry
Bone profile	Hepatitis A screening
Stool examination	Spirometry
Thyroid screen	Hepatitis B screening
Cervical smear	Chest X-ray
Full cholesterol profile	Rheumatoid factor
Vision tests	ECG
Liver function tests	Venereal disease
Tonometry	Cardiac stress test
Kidney function tests	HIV screen
Retinal camera	

UK cost (approx): £350–1,000
See Section Two: Belgium; Costa Rica; Hungary;
India; Malaysia; Poland;
South Africa; Thailand

Chapter Ten

TRANSPLANT SURGERY

Transplant surgery is the most serious of all procedures, because often it's the patient's last hope and donors must be found to facilitate the treatment going ahead. More than 1,500 kidney transplants are performed in the UK every year, but there could be many more if more donors were found. It is the same with other transplants. If there were more donors, more operations could take place.

Fortunately, transplant surgeons are highly skilled and techniques are continually improving to a degree where, while a transplant is not as routine as, say, a tonsillectomy, there are very high success rates in all areas with patients surviving for a long time and leading a normal life afterwards.

KIDNEYS
We have two kidneys; they are located at the back of the body, are bean-shaped and are about the size of a fist. They are very important because they clean the blood

and remove waste products. They also help make red blood cells, control blood pressure, and balance water and salt in the body.

When the kidneys fail due to illness or injury, they stop filtering and cleaning properly, which can affect the heart, lungs, brain and other organs and can eventually lead to death.

There are three treatment options: hemodialysis, peritoneal dialysis and kidney transplantation. For some patients a transplant is the only answer and it gives a better quality of life with more freedom than having to be hooked up to a dialysis machine, and there is also a noted increase in energy levels.

There are two types of transplant: those that come from a living donor who may be a family member, close friend or even a stranger, and those from an unrelated donor who has died – a non-living donor. Surveys show that, after 10 to 15 years, 50 per cent of transplanted kidneys are still functional and those from living relatives do better than those from non-living donors.

The actual operation is performed under a general anaesthetic and takes between two and three hours. An incision about eight to ten inches long is made in the abdomen. The blood supply of the new kidney is attached to the patient's blood supply and the ureter attached to the bladder. The old kidneys are left in place and the new one located in the pelvic region.

The most important complication after surgery is that the kidney might be rejected by the body's immune system, which guards against attack by foreign matter. This is overcome by medication, which has to be taken every day to combat rejection. Post-operative patients are usually put on a special diet, but they may find this less restrictive than the one they were advised to follow if they were previously on dialysis.

UK cost (approx):   £25,000+; annual
                     immunosuppression
                     drugs £5,000+
See Section Two: Costa Rica; India; Israel;
                     South Africa

HEART

Congestive heart failure is a frightening disease where the patient is unable to walk and finds it very difficult to breathe, and it may be that the best option is a transplant. Sadly, there is a worldwide shortage of donor hearts, which are removed only when a doctor certifies a person 'brain dead'.

The heart transplant is one of the most remarkable procedures in modern medicine. A team of surgeons open up the chest of the patient, who is then connected to an artificial heart and lung machine that keeps the blood circulating. While the damaged heart is being removed at the patient's hospital, the second (donor) heart is also removed and kept in a cold chemical solution. It is usually airlifted by helicopter to the patient's hospital where it is sewn into place and the blood vessels connected. As the new heart begins to warm up, it starts to beat, although sometimes an electric shock may be needed. After everything is checked for leaks, the patient is disconnected from the artificial heart and lung machine. The whole operation can take up to six hours, depending on the patient's medical history.

There will be a stay for up to three days in an intensive care unit at the hospital, and the patient will be given anti-rejection medication. The whole hospital stay should not be more than about 14 days. The 'miracle' is that the patient will immediately feel the difference made by the healthy heart.

Post-operative patients will be expected to make lifestyle changes to look after their new heart. Caffeine, alcohol and tobacco are out, and a progressive daily exercise programme is vital for full recovery and to rebuild muscle strength.

UK cost (approx): £70,000+
See Section Two: Costa Rica; India; Israel;
                   South Africa

LIVER

The liver is the largest organ in the body, located on the right side of the abdomen behind the lower ribs and below the lungs. It keeps the body healthy with more than 400 functions a day. It removes toxic substances like alcohol, makes proteins for blood clotting and stores vitamins, fats, iron and sugars for later use, to name just a few.

The first full liver transplant was performed as far back as 1964. There are many reasons why patients may need a new liver, from alcohol-induced cirrhosis to hepatitis sufferers and people with cystic fibrosis.

Instead of a patient waiting for a full liver from a non-living donor, sometimes a living donor can give a portion of their liver to a recipient. This was first demonstrated in the United States in 1989 when a mother gave a segment of her liver to her child. The liver grows to full size in six to eight weeks.

A full liver transplant operation usually lasts between six and eight hours, but it can take longer. The central process involves joining the patient's blood vessels and bile duct to the donor liver, after first totally removing the diseased one. The abdominal incision is shaped like an upside down 'Y', and for a brief period of time during the operation the patient is without a liver at all.

The stay in hospital can vary considerably but is usually around three weeks. As with all transplant surgery, the patient is given anti-rejection drugs and a biopsy is usually taken a week after surgery to see how well the liver is working.

Again, lifestyle changes have to be made to accommodate the new liver. If the liver was necessary because of cirrhosis, then, obviously, boozing is out.

UK cost (approx):   £75,000+
See Section Two: Costa Rica; India; Israel;
                   South Africa

PANCREAS

The pancreas is a gland situated near the stomach that secretes a digestive fluid into the intestine through one or more ducts, and also secretes the hormone insulin. Candidates for a pancreas transplant are diabetics with Type 1 diabetes who need to improve blood sugar control, whether or not they have had a kidney transplant earlier or need to have both transplants at once.

The healthy pancreas comes from a person who has been declared 'brain dead' but remains on life support. It is transported to the recipient in a cooled solution that preserves the pancreas for up to 20 hours. It is then implanted in the right lower portion of the patient's abdomen, but the diseased pancreas is not removed. Insulin from the transplanted pancreas is released into the bloodstream through the veins in the lower abdomen.

The operation is done only in hospitals that also do kidney transplants, and often the two procedures are carried out at the same time. After a pancreas transplant, the patient will have to take anti-rejection drugs, to suppress the immune system, for the rest of their life, but many people who have a successful transplant find they may no longer have the symptoms or need to treat diabetes.

TRANSPLANT SURGERY

UK cost (approx):   £35,000+
See Section Two: India; Israel; South Africa

LUNG

Some chronic illnesses, like emphysema, can cause destruction of the lung tissue, while others, such as pulmonary fibrosis, can result in the lung being scarred and oxygen levels depleted. Diseases like bronchiectasis and cystic fibrosis may cause chronic infection. In all cases, they can be effectively treated with a lung transplant, and most patients may only require one new lung.

Lungs have to be donated from someone who has been declared 'brain dead', and recipients usually have to undergo a bank of medical tests to make sure they are appropriate for a transplant. Because, as with all transplants, there is a serious shortage of donors, some recipients may have to wait months or even years before they can have an operation.

The operation is one of the longest, with a single lung transplant taking anything up to eight hours; when both lungs are transplanted, it might take 12 hours.

The chest cavity is opened, with an incision across the entire chest underneath the breasts if a double-lung transplant is required. The damaged lung or lungs are removed and the donor lungs placed in the chest cavity, with the surgeon connecting the blood vessels to and from the lung and main airway.

Post-operative patients are moved to an intensive care

unit for a few days, where they are hooked up to a breathing tube and mechanical ventilator. The total time in hospital depends on the patient, but is usually around two weeks.

After the transplant, the patient must not smoke at all for the rest of his or her life, allow only a very small alcohol intake and make sure their diet is highly nutritious.

UK cost (approx): heart and lung £100,000+
See Section Two: India; Israel; South Africa

SECTION TWO

INTRODUCTION

Making a decision about something as important as your own health obviously should not be done lightly, and many factors need to be taken into consideration. When that decision involves going abroad for elective surgery, then a few additional concerns may need to be mulled over.

Many people might dismiss out of hand having surgery abroad, from some sort of misplaced idea that anything 'foreign' can't possibly be as good as the treatment they would receive in the UK. A fairly healthy cynicism is always a good thing to have, but too much narrow-mindedness means patients are often ruling out some of the most highly advanced medical centres in the world for the supposed safety of ageing and overcrowded British hospitals.

The most important thing to do if you take the step of travelling abroad for treatment is to research thoroughly the destinations and establishments you may wish to go to, and be realistic about your expectations. That is where this guide comes in.

The hospitals and centres mentioned in the following section of this book all have contact details – usually their Internet web-based address, their telephone number, their email address and the actual address of the establishment. These facts are your most important first port of call.

If you have an Internet connection at home, then obviously it is quite easy to enter the URL in your browser and find out more about the establishment of your choice. Any specific questions you have can be sent to them by email and the whole process is a lot swifter than corresponding by ordinary mail.

But even if you don't have a computer, there will be one with Internet access available at your local library free of charge, where you will also be able to print out information. Or, if that is not convenient, then you may be able to use a nearby Internet café.

If Internet use is completely out of the question, you may wish to send the hospital a letter, or phone the establishment, which will usually have an English-speaking person with whom you can talk.

Whatever approach you decide to use, make sure you research thoroughly as many establishments as possible in your chosen destination, to make sure they perform the exact procedure that you require.

Remember to elicit testimonials from all the establishments you approach and don't take them merely at face value. They will obviously send you only ones that praise their centre so do ask for the name, address and telephone number of the person making the testimonial – and get in touch with them personally to find out exactly what they thought and if they had any qualms at all about their treatment. Also remember that reputations of establishments can vary from year to year, so make sure the testimonials you do get are the most up-to-date, and not something that was written 10 years ago.

The most important consideration when it comes to your medical procedure is the treatment itself. This may sound obvious, but do keep it in mind. While it might be a fantastic idea to whisk yourself off to a fabulous exotic location where you can recuperate while dipping your toes into crystal-clear warm waters or strolling along a pristine white beach, make sure the nearby medical establishment also meets your discerning needs. Don't compromise at all in this area. It might mean you have to settle for a clinic in Europe on a drizzling winter's day, but at least you won't have to live to regret it.

That's not to say that some facilities in far-flung places like India, Costa Rica, South Africa and Thailand are not equal to Western establishments – many surpass them in terms of world-class technical excellence, and are staffed by the very best accomplished surgeons. Just make sure the one you choose really is the one for you. The emphasis in 'medical tourism' should be more on the *medical* and less on the *tourism*. The tropics are wonderful, but the climate can also be very hot and humid and, while hospitals, clinics and hotels will all be air-conditioned, sightseeing can be much more tiring than in temperate lands

And then there is the price – Wherever you choose to go and whichever procedure you choose to have, the cost – including your post-operative holiday – will be substantially less than the average private hospital cost of the operation alone in the UK. The prices given in this guide are as accurate as possible at the time of publication, but they are liable to change at any time. One of the main factors for price change, apart from fluctuations in market rates and inflation, is that the medical needs for each individual patient are different. A final price can be given only by the hospital, medical centre or UK agent, once they are aware of all the treatment that will be involved in a particular case.

While cost is one of the major reasons for the rise in medical tourism over the last decade, there are still one or two other factors to consider. India, with its glittering, high-tech Apollo Hospitals, offers dirt-cheap operations compared with the UK. But you will have to factor in the cost of the return air flight. With economy flights to all the major subcontinent cities at little more than £500 return, this may not seem to be an issue. But remember the journey is long – around nine hours. After surgery, do you really want to spend that length of time cramped in economy class with little leg space, or would you rather pay substantially more for the comfort of stretching out in business class? If a friend or partner is accompanying you, then the potential cost of two business class seats has to be taken into consideration for all long-haul destinations.

Unless you feel that your surgery is absolutely urgent, remember to allow yourself a few days to acclimatise to your new surroundings before going into hospital and, even more importantly, allow plenty of time for your post-operative recuperation holiday. Your clinic or medical adviser will tell you what they think is the minimum time you should spend before you are able to travel back to the UK, but it is always a good idea to add on a few more days so that your homeward journey is even more comfortable.

Many hospitals and clinics outside Europe that are featured in this guide boast that their surgeons are trained in the West – many in the UK itself. Satisfy yourself that this really is the case and that their qualifications are up to scratch. Find out who your surgeon will be and, if possible, deal with him or her personally.

And don't forget to inform the person from whom you buy your travel insurance that you are travelling to have medical treatment. This may, or may not, affect the premium you pay or nullify any clauses in the policy.

Also mention the subject of your travel to your doctor, or anyone who may be giving you inoculations for your long-haul travel or a prescription for malaria tablets. And inform your surgeon on or before arrival of the inoculations or tablets you are taking. It is doubtful any of them will interfere with your surgery but your mind will be at rest.

Bon Voyage.

DESTINATIONS COVERED

ARGENTINA

OFFICIAL NAME: Republica de Argentina
AREA: 2,766,890 square kilometres
(1,068,302 square miles)
POPULATION: 39,537,943
LANGUAGE: Spanish
CAPITAL: Buenos Aires
TIME ZONE: Three hours behind Greenwich Mean Time
(GMT −3)
DISTANCE: London to Buenos Aires = 11,161
kilometres (6,920 miles)

ARGENTINA'S European-styled capital city Buenos Aires has long been acknowledged as one of the leading world centres for elective cosmetic surgery as well as dentistry and ophthalmology. Due to the economic policies of the 1990s, when parity was established between the Argentine peso and the American dollar, hospitals in the South American country were able to upgrade to the very latest technological equipment. It means world-class centres for medical tourists who come mainly from Europe and the USA.

These centres include:

ARGENTINE ACADEMY OF COSMETIC SURGERY
It has two operating theatres and rooms with five beds for patient recovery. It covers all areas of cosmetic

surgery and specialises in cellulites and localised obesity treatments as well as face rejuvenation and laser treatments.

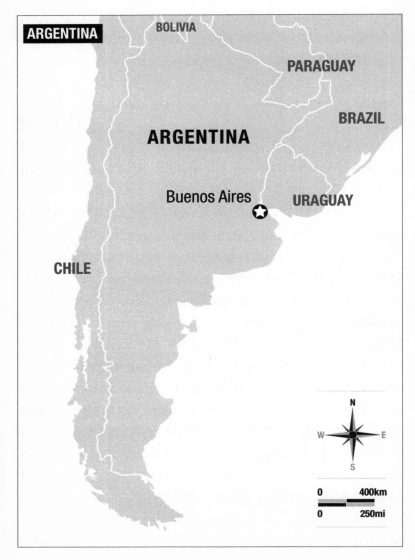

ROBLES CLINIC OF PLASTIC SURGERY
Virrey del Pino 2530, Capital Federal, Argentina
Tel: +54 11 4784 8393
Under the direction of the world-renowned Dr Jose M
Robles, a specialist in reconstructive and plastic surgery,
it has state-of-the-art operating theatres and was
established in 1983.

THE DENTISTRY CLINIC
Run by Dr Norberto Coerezza, the clinic has four dental
offices, operating room, sterilisation room and dental
lab. It is the clinic chosen and approved by the American
and Canadian Embassies in Argentina for the treatment
of its personnel and American residents in Buenos Aires
and the rest of Latin America.

HAIR RECOVERY ARGENTINA
Avenue Córdoba 827, Pisos 1ro y 2do,
Buenos Aires, Argentina
Tel/Fax: +54 11 4311 1025
Email: info@hairrecovery.com.ar
Specialises in micro-graft hair transplants and is
dedicated to the study and treatment of baldness. It has
special rooms for digital photography, which lets
doctors, alongside patients, design future looks
according to physical features, original hair colour and
other criteria.

KAUFER EYE CLINIC

Carlos Pellegrini 2266, B1640BNT, Martínez,
Prov. de Buenos Aires, Argentina
Tel: +54 11 4733 0560/4563
Email: info@kaufer.com

Specialises in all eye-surgery techniques, and is especially proficient in cataracts. The team keeps up-to-date with the most recent worldwide advances through scientific papers, conferences and congresses.

THE GYNAECOLOGY AND FERTILITY INSTITUTE

Founded in 1985 for the needs of infertile couples, the Institute provides assistance by using ultrasound diagnoses, laboratory exams and surgical treatments.

Since December 2001 and the devaluation of the Argentine peso, the country has become a much more affordable place to visit. Because of the vast size of the country – second only to Brazil in South America – medical tourists usually restrict their tourism to Buenos Aires and its surrounding areas. The capital itself is a modern and dynamic city considered by many to be the 'pearl' of South America. The immediate impact of its European architecture, reminiscent of Paris, is stunning. Add to that the vibrancy of its people, who seem to be obsessed with the tango and football, and you have a heady mix. Nightclubs, discos and bars are open until the very early hours and because of the city's agreeable temperatures all year round (mean annual temperature

18 degrees centigrade) visitors can walk around the city in any season. July is the coldest month in winter, but frosts are infrequent and a woollen coat and scarf are sufficient when going out. In summer (December to February), the mean temperature is 28 degrees centigrade and coats are not needed. Rains are more frequent in autumn and spring.

Walking the avenues of Buenos Aires is the best way to enjoy this city. Although there is no defining tourist landmark – like the Eiffel Tower in Paris or the Empire State Building in New York – many of the old buildings are breathtaking to look at and beautifully preserved.

Worth seeing is The Cabildo of Buenos Aires, which once worked as a city hall and was built in 1764. It was where Spain gave independence to Argentina in 1810 and is now a museum situated opposite Plaza de Mayo between Bolivar Street and Avenida de Mayo. The 67.5m (222ft) Obelisco was built in 1936 to celebrate 400 years of the founding of Buenos Aires. It's on the crossroads of 9 de Julio and Corrientes Avenues. There are 206 steps up to the top to get an excellent view of the city from the obelisk's four windows.

Other buildings to see are Government House, also known as the Pink House, built in 1580, and the Cathedral at Avenidas Rivadavia and San Martin among many others.

When you are fed up with the museums and historical places, walk along the Avenida de Mayo or pop into one of the city's famous coffee houses situated on Avenida 9 de Julio. And then in the evening go to a tango show in San Telmo or to one of the live rock and jazz clubs that dot the city.

PACKAGES

Plenitas, who are based in Buenos Aires (www.plenitas.com), offer package deals that combine medical treatments with tourism and include hotel accommodation. Lodging is usually at the four-star Cabildo Suites Apart Hotel, located in the main centre of the Belgrano district near the subway, cinemas and shopping centres. It has 24-hour room service, coffee shop, spa and gym. The rooms include cable TV, air-conditioning, microwave, minibar, Internet, safe box, tableware and kitchenette.

All packages include transfers to and from the airport as well as to the clinics for appointments plus the use of a personal bilingual assistant. They do NOT include flights to Buenos Aires.

Here are examples of some of the treatments available:

Nose surgery £915 ($1,739) All treatment and 7 nights at Cabildo Suites
Silicon breast implants £1,437 ($2,732)
All treatment and 10 nights at Cabildo Suites
Fertility treatment £3,218 ($6,115) Including ovulation stimulation and insemination plus 20 nights at the Cabildo Suites

Facial lifting £1,114 ($2,139) Can also include a
cervicoplasty, which treats the neck area, plus 8
nights at the Cabildo Suites

Laser eye surgery one eye £734 ($1,395);
both eyes £1,260 ($2,395) Treatment plus 5 nights
at Cabildo Suites

Liposuction £734 ($1,395) Removal of fat tissue
plus five nights at Cabildo Suites

Complete cosmetic dental treatment £5,336
($10,140) Includes 8 full porcelain crowns; 6
porcelain full metal crowns; 14 root canal
treatments; 8 fibreglass posts; 6 metal posts; 10
provisional crowns, and 14 nights at Cabildo Suites

Plenitas offer many more packages including tummy
tucks, chin implants and penis lengthening, plus the
opportunity to create your own package. You can
contact them through their website or by calling +54 11
6348 2833.

Louis William Rose from Jacksonville, Florida, decided
to have his dental surgery with Plenitas in the
Argentinean capital of Buenos Aries.

He says, 'When I first considered using Plenitas for
dental implants, I naturally had some reservations. I
knew nothing about their company, they were located in
a country that I had never visited, and I did not speak
the language. However, after checking the references
that they gave me, I made the decision to go. I am so

glad that I did. The dental treatment and facilities are of the highest quality and employ the latest technology. The personal care and service that I received from the Plenitas account executive assigned to me made me feel completely assured and at home. And what a wonderful city Buenos Aires is!'

HOTELS

For independent travellers wanting to set up their own treatment at one of the clinics, there is a vast array of hotels available in Buenos Aires in all price ranges.

Five star: Four Seasons Hotel in the exclusive Le Recoleta district (www.fourseasons.com/buenosaires). Price £80–160 per night.

Sheraton Libertador in the downtown district (www.sheraton.com/libertador). Price £55–160 per night.

Four star: Park Plaza Kempinski in the heart of Recoleta (www.parkplazahotels.com/plaza_ingles/index.htm). Price £55–80 per night.

Hotel Republica in downtown (www.hotelrepublica.com.ar/start.swf). Price £27–55 per night.

Bed and Breakfast: Caseron Porteno, small six-room guesthouse in the Palermo neighbourhood (www.caseronporteno.com). Price £13–26 per night.

FARES

Flights from London to Buenos Aires start from around £500 return in economy class with a choice of airlines including Air France, United Airlines and Lufthansa.

The first person to perform a heart bypass on a patient suffering from coronary heart disease was Argentinean Dr Rene Geronimo Favaloro, who created the technique in 1967. Although Dr Favaloro was working in the United States at the time, he returned to Argentina in 1971 and established the Favaloro Foundation, which is one of the largest institutions dedicated to cardiology in Latin America.

BELGIUM

OFFICIAL NAME: Kingdom of Belgium
AREA: 32,820 square kilometres (12,672 square miles)
POPULATION: 10,339,000
LANGUAGES: Dutch, French, German
CAPITAL: Brussels
TIME ZONE: Central European Time (GMT +1)
DISTANCE: London to Brussels = 349 kilometres
(217 miles)

Belgium is at the forefront of medical tourism and is one of the major European countries encouraging overseas private patients. It's not difficult to see why. There is a high quality of treatment within the Belgian healthcare system and it has the lowest post-operative infection rates in Europe. Waiting times for surgery are seven to 14 days and, because of the independent status of Belgian hospitals, all revenues are ploughed back into new equipment allowing them to have the very latest tools. For instance, there are 12 Positon Emission Tomography (PET) scanners for cancer detection in Belgium as against four in the UK at the time of writing.

But the thing that clinches treatment in Belgium for most medical tourists is the cost. It is a fraction of what you would pay for private treatment in Britain and yet is only a few hours away by Eurostar. Virtually all medical staff speak English and you have access to English TV.

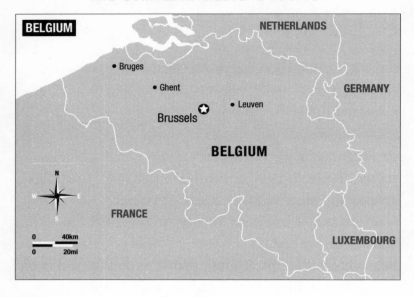

Belgium is becoming so popular with patients that UK companies have been set up to manage the growth industry, offering door-to-door service.

DIRECT HEALTHCARE INTERNATIONAL LTD

26 York Street, London W1U 6PZ, UK

Tel: 020 7553 3421

Email: info@direct-healthcare.com

Can arrange everything from hip replacement, knee replacement, hip resurfacing, gastric banding and cosmetic surgery (liposuction, breast augmentation, breast enlargement, breast reduction) to heart-bypass surgery and prostate surgery. They have a number of useful websites: www.direct-healthcare.com; www.total-hip-replacement-surgery.com; www.quality-cosmetic-surgery.com; www.knee-replacement-surgery.co.uk.

ORTHOPAEDIC

Their all-inclusive prices include pick-up and return from point of arrival in Belgium and the hospital they use for orthopaedic surgery is located near the city of Bruges. It boasts the latest technology with a staff of more than 400 and 40 physicians. The hospital places a strong emphasis on cleanliness and the quality of food. All meals are prepared on site and the menu changes daily. The hospital accommodation varies depending on the medical procedure undertaken and whether you choose to be in a shared or single room. Usually there are two people to a room but, for a supplement, single rooms are available.

Their prices are:

Hip arthroscopy: £1,400 (€2,038) Stay: 2 days

Total hip replacement: £5,600 (€8,099)
   Stay: 11 days

Hip revision: £8,500 (€12,292) Stay: 16 days

Hip resurfacing (Birmingham hip): £6,025 (€8,769)
   Stay: 11 days

Bilateral hip replacement (double hip): £11,200
(€16,198) Stay: 22 days

Knee arthroscopy: £1,400 (€2,038) Stay: 1 day

Bilateral knee arthroscopy: £2,800 (€4,075)
   Stay: 2 days

Total knee replacement: £6,500 (€9,400)
   Stay: 13 days

Knee revision: £9,700 (€14,118) Stay: 14 days

Bilateral knee replacement: £12,950 (€18,922)
   Stay: 24 days

Oxford knee replacement (half knee):
   £6,500 (€9,400) Stay: 9 days
Cruciate ligament reconstruction: £3,450 (€5,022)
   Stay: 6 days

COSMETIC SURGERY

The cosmetic surgery clinic is located in Leuven and is the most modern in Belgium. It is newly completed and boasts state-of-the-art, 3D camera-assisted surgery. Surgeon Dr Wim de Maerteleire is especially known for the quality of his breast uplifts.

Prices quoted are an approximate guide only, as each person is different and therefore each treatment slightly differs.

Botox injection (first area): £250 (€365)
Botox (next area), glabellar furrows, forehead wrinkles, crows' feet: £190 (€278)
Breast enlargement, high-profile cohesive silicon gel-filled implants with textured surfacing: £3,469 (€4,995)
Anatomical implants: £3,937 (€5,670)
Mini breast lift: £1,594 (€2,295)
Scarless mini breast with laser: £2,812 (4,050)
Breast lift with internal muscle bra fixation: £3,844 (€5,535)
Breast reduction: £3,468 (€4,995)
Buttock implants: £3,658 (€5,205)
Ear surgery: £1,200 (€1,460)
EYELID SURGERY
Upper eyelids: £1,125 (€1,620)

Lower eyelids: £1,312 (€ 1,890)

Upper and lower eyelids: £1,969 (€ 2,835)

FACIAL SURGERY

Mini facelift (Macs-lift or S-lift): £3,281 (4,725)

Mini facelift and upper eyelids: £3,937 (€ 5670)

Mini facelift and lower eyelids: £4,125 (€ 5940)

Mini facelift plus upper and lower eyelids:
£4,687 (€ 6,750)

Neck correction: £2,065 (€ 2,973)

Mini facelift and neck correction: £3,881 (€ 5,589)

Mini facelift, neck correction plus upper and lower
eyelids: £5,487 (€ 7,901)

Forehead lift: £2,719 (€ 2,920)

Forehead lift (endoscopic): £3,187 (€ 4,590)

Brow lift: £1,025 (€ 1,497)

Lip enhancement: £375-625 (€ 547-913)

Nose reshaping (tip correction): £2,812 (€ 4,050)

Total nose reshaping: £3,750 (€ 5,400)

LIPOSUCTION

1-2 areas, local anaesthesia: £1,125 (€ 1,620)

1-2 areas, general anaesthesia: £1,687 (€ 2,430)

2-3 areas, general anaesthesia: £2,062 (€ 2,970)

3-4 areas, general anaesthesia: £2,062 (€ 2,970)

OTHER

Gynaecomasty: £3,300 (€ 4,818)

Male chest enhancement, both pectoral
implants included: £5,350 (€ 7,811)

Nipple correction: £875 (€ 1,278)

Mini tummy tuck (abdominoplasty),

below midriff or naval: £2,344 (€3,375)
Full tummy tuck, above and below
midriff or naval: £2,906 (€4,185)

The company will also arrange obesity surgery under Dr Dillemans, who has carried out 3,500 procedures and is Belgium's leading surgeon in the field.

Paediatric heart surgery is carried out in Ghent University Hospital, while cardiac surgery is carried out in Germany at the heart centre in Lahr, which boasts an excellent reputation and has been used by royalty. Eye surgery is carried out by Professor Dr Jean Assaf, head of eye surgery at St Pierre Hospital, Basilk Hospital and Brussels Eye Centre, while wrist and ankle surgery is under the supervision of Dr Kris Beudts St Michel's in Brussels, an expert in micro orthopaedic surgery. For the cost of any of these procedures, or any other treatment, contact Direct Healthcare International Ltd. The prices do NOT include fares to and from Belgium.

CLINIC BEAUCARE
(www.kliniekbeaucare.com/belgium/clinic_beaucare.html)
Peutiesesteenweg 111, B-1830 Machelen, Brussels
Tel: +32 2 756 0404 Fax: +32 2 756 0405
Email: contact@kliniekbeaucare.com
Can arrange a consultation in London on the type of cosmetic surgery you want, but you will have to arrange your own travel to Belgium. Clinic

Beaucare's website contains plenty of travel and hotel information.

The clinic practises only cosmetic surgery and with all operations patients can leave the clinic the same day.

Their prices are:

Lifting inner thigh: £2,450
Lifting buttock: £1,850
Armlift: £1,550
Botox injection for first area: £200
Botox injection for next area: £100
Salt-water breast implants: £1,960
High-profile cohesive gel silicone-filled breast implants with textured surfacing: £1,960–2,200
Anatomical breast implants: £2,720
Breast reduction: £2,300–2,900
Breast uplift without implant: £2,120–2,850
Breast uplift with implants: £2,700–3,450
Buttock implants: £2,850
Chin enlargement with implant: £1,550
Ear reshaping: £900
Upper-eyelid surgery: £1,050
Lower-eyelid surgery: £1,150
Upper and lower eyelids: £1,600
FACELIFT
Mini facelift (S-lift): £1,650–2,250
Mini facelift and upper eyelids: £2,550
Mini facelift and lower eyelids: £2,650

Mini facelift plus upper and lower eyelids: £2,950

Neck correction: £1,650

Mini facelift and neck correction: £2,950

Mini facelift, neck correction plus upper and
lower eyelids: £3,350–3,750

Forehead lift: £1,600

Brow lift: £820

OTHER

Labia reduction: £1,280

Lip enhancement: £650

Gynaecomastia: £1,550

Nose reshaping/rhinoplasty: £1,650–2,850

Nose tip: £1,050

Mini abdominoplasty: £1,400

Full tummy tuck: £1,780–2,350

Belgium is often overlooked as a tourist destination because it is either thought of as too near to the UK to be exotic, too boring because of its European Union connections, or because it is overshadowed by its huge neighbour, France. But in fact Belgium can be quite enchanting and, because of its compact size, easy to get around.

The image of Brussels is one of faceless bureaucracy, but, in fact, its central square, the Grand'Place, is lined with exuberantly impressive and ornate guild houses focused on the Gothic heights of the Hotel de Ville and is anything but faceless. It is the centre of the city's social and civic life and is famous for its café/bars and its

Sunday-morning bird market. There is nothing better in the Grand'Place than sitting around sipping a Stella Artois beer and people watching.

The Royal Palace and the House of Parliament lie to the east of the Grand'Place on higher ground, and in between there is a formal park. Every area of Brussels has its own distinctive market, whether it's horse flesh, cheeses or chickens, antiques or flowers. And don't forget to taste the famous Belgian chocolates as well as the mussels.

Bruges is the most visited town in Belgium and it's like going back in time about 500 years because it has Europe's best medieval buildings. It is so stunning that many people think it's 'fake'; in some ways they are right because 19th-century neo-gothic style is more prevalent than you might think. But don't let that spoil a visit to a remarkable town. It's packed with tourists in the summer but many are on day trips, so the trick is to stay overnight and enjoy the quieter nightlife.

Traces of the Middle Ages are also found in Ghent, especially around the old port with its guild halls on the Graslei and Korenlei. Another attraction is the medieval fortress of the Count of Flanders. There is also a lively nightlife in Ghent with welcoming bars throughout the heart of the town.

Antwerp is Belgium's second largest city with a population of more than 500,000. Just think of the name Antwerp and you think of diamonds; the diamond district around the railway station is well worth exploring. While the city doesn't have the 'wow' factor of Bruges, there are plenty of monuments to admire and numerous paintings by Rubens, who lived there in the 17th century.

FARES

Return fares to Brussels on Eurostar start from as little as £120 in standard class to £410 in business class. Return bucket-shop flights are around £100.

Package deal medical-tourist specialists can arrange for any family and friends to stay in hotels near to where the procedure is taking place. If you want to arrange your own accommodation or tour the country after your treatment, then be prepared to pay around £30 (€45) per night for modest accommodation to more than £100 (€150) for first-class accommodation. And remember that in summer all the major tourist towns are full so it is best to book well ahead.

The law on voluntary euthanasia came into force in Belgium on 23 September 2002 subject to prescribed conditions:

- The patient is an adult or emancipated minor, capable and conscious at the time of his or her request;
- The request is made voluntarily, is well thought out and reiterated, and is not the result of outside pressure;
- The patient is in a hopeless medical condition and complains of constant and unbearable physical or mental pain which cannot be relieved.

COSTA RICA

OFFICIAL NAME: Republic of Costa Rica
AREA: 51,100 square kilometres (19,730 square miles)
POPULATION: 4,016,173
LANGUAGE: Spanish
CAPITAL: San José
TIME ZONE: Six hours behind Greenwich Mean Time (GMT –6)
DISTANCE: London to San José = 8,719 kilometres (5,418 miles)

Costa Rica is a Central American country famed for its natural beauty and has been a neutral nation since 1948 when it disbanded its army. It is a major tourist destination, especially for Americans, and has built up a high reputation for medical tourism.

COSTA RICA HEALTH GATEWAYS

(www.costaricahealthgateways.com)
Apdo, 293-Plaza Colonial, Escazu, Costa Rica
Tel: +506 203 0145 Fax: +506 282 6181
Email: feelgood@costaricahealthgateways.com
Specialises in both cosmetic and dental treatments. It has bilingual staff and your stay may be in three different locations around the country.

For cosmetic procedures, the company uses CIMA Hospital, Hospital Clinica Catolica, and the Peralta

Clinic of Plastic and Aesthetic Surgery in San José. For dental treatment, they use Gil Clinic San Pedro on the east side of San José City and Gil Clinic Escazu on the west side. They accept Visa, Master Card and American Express credit cards.

ACCOMMODATION PACKAGES
(Prices quoted here exclude any treatment costs)
At Santa Ana (Sun Valley), Costa Rica Health Gateways offers a standard non-air-conditioned room package at $120 (£67) a day which includes all meals, snacks, beverages, post-operative care plus airport and clinic transportation. Non-surgical accompanying guests are charged $60 (£34) a day. For $140 (£78), there is an upgrade to a larger room with air-conditioning and view, and a $180 (£100) per day deluxe package gets the

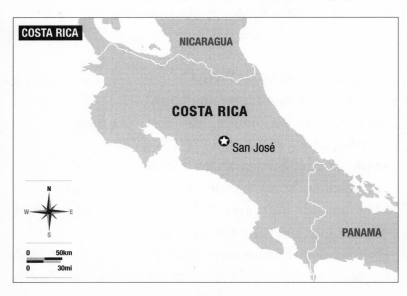

standard package plus air-conditioned room, cocktails, unlimited spa use, daily massage, manicure and pedicure, laundry services and internet access. Accompanying non-surgical guests are charged $70 (£39) per day.

A second package in San Antonio de Belen with bed and breakfast and an onsite staff nurse costs $85 (£47) a day or $50 (£28) for a non-surgical guest. For full board, snacks and access to a one-day tour, the price rises to $105 (£58). The lodging in San Antonio de Belen boasts a swimming pool and two acres of landscaped gardens.

A third package in Escazu offers the usual transportation to clinics and to and from the airport plus full board for $95 (£53) a day. Deluxe rooms are $105 (£59) with mini-suites at $115 (£64) and non-surgical guests get a discount of around 40 per cent.

COSMETIC
The company emphasises that prices vary depending on each person's body condition.

Facelift: $3,000–4,700 (£1,667–2,611)
Eyelid surgery: $1,200–1,800 (£667–1,000)
Neck lift: $1,600–2,000 (£889–1,111)
Liposuction: $700–3,600 (£389–2,000)
Arm tuck: $2,100–3,000 (£1,167–2,000)
Ear surgery: $1,200–1,800 (£667–1,000)
Nose surgery: $1,900–3,500 (£1,056–1,944)
Cheek implants: $1,200–1,800 (£667–1,000)

Chin implants: $1,200–2,200 (£667–1,222)
Breast augmentation: $2,800–3,500 (£1,556–1,944)
Breast reduction: $2,900–3,900 (£1,611–2,167)
Tummy tuck: $3,000–4,100 (£1,667–2,278)
Buttock implants: $3,000–5,200 (£1,667–2,889)
Fat grafting: $1,200–3,800 (£667–2,111)

Costa Rica Health Gateways can also arrange complete medical check-ups at a fraction of the cost of those in the UK. They range from the basic traveller package to the deluxe package, which includes:

Comprehensive medical history and physical examination (including pelvic exam with cervical smear for women)

Hearing test

Lab test to include: complete blood count, comprehensive metabolic panels for electrolytes

Glaucoma test detection

Lung-functions test

Electrocardiogram

Kidney and liver function

Glucose test for diabetes

Cholesterol test

Urinalysis

Other tests include blood tests to measure iron level, peptic ulcer disease, prostate cancer, female hormone assessment (for women who are concerned about menopause) and a confidential HIV test as well as hepatitis and thyroid tests.

Imaging tests to include: X-ray, electron beam scan (heart-disease detection), abdominal ultrasound, mammogram, and osteoporosis and stroke exam.

Examination of the lower part of the colon and rectum to detect polyps and early cancer.

Immunisations to include: flu shot, diphtheria, tetanus, polio, measles, mumps and rubella, as well as a tuberculosis skin test.

PRISMA DENTAL
(www.cosmetics-dentistry.com)
Rhomoser Boulevard, Banco Uno, 3rd floor,
San José, Costa Rica
Tel: +506 291 5151 Fax: +506 291 5454
Email: dental@cosmetics-dentistry.com
Also offer dental packages for the medical tourist. They offer all dental treatment including implants and veneers, and can also assist with accommodation.

MEZA DENTAL CARE
(www.mezadentalcare.com)
Clinica Hospital Santa Catalina, San José, Costa Rica
Tel: +506 305 6392
Email: info@mezadentalcare.com
Established in 1990 and specialise in every dental procedure. The company designs special medical-tourist packages in which the patient is met at the airport and the stay in Costa Rica is co-ordinated with the dental surgery. A representative is available throughout the

stay to assist with any needs the patient may have. All representatives speak Spanish and English and the clinic is only 25 minutes away from San José Airport.

Here are some of the prices for dental treatment only. For package deals, email the company:

Consultation:	$30 (£17)

X-RAYS

Periapical:	$20 (£12)
Diagnosis set (6):	$90 (£50)
Panoramic:	$50 (£28)

SURGERY

Wisdom teeth:	from $250 (£139)
Tooth extraction:	$60 (£34)
Implant surgery:	$700 (£389)
Root canal (1 canal):	$150 (£84)
Root canal (2 canal):	$200 (£112)
Root canal (3 or more canals):	$275
Ultrasonic cleaning:	$85 (£47)
Cleaning (polishing):	$55 (£30)
Total denture (each):	$500 (£278)
Partial denture:	$550 (£305)
Base metal crown:	$200 (£112)
Base metal porcelain crown:	$250 (£139)
High nobel metal porcelain crown:	$400 (£222)
Porcelain crown:	$350 (£195)
Gold crown:	$400 (£222)
Endo post:	$150 (£84)
Porcelain veneer:	$300 (£167)
Bleaching:	$300 (£167)

Costa Rica's dry season runs from December to April, when the country is at its hottest, with heavy tropical rains from May to October. In December and January, the north and northeast trade winds blow, bringing down temperatures in the late afternoon and evening.

The country boasts excellent beaches and great surfing with luxury resorts and deserted coves on the Pacific coast. The Caribbean coast has national parks and wildlife refuges with conservation areas for turtle breeding. The whole county is eco-conscious, with lush jungles that are packed with monkeys, crocodiles and exotic birds.

When landing in San José, you might be surprised to see how 'American' it is, with its fast-food outlets and department stores. But it also has colourful markets, good museums and a fine climate.

Costa Ricans have a laid-back attitude to living, which makes them very friendly, but if you get fed up with kicking back there is deep-sea diving to experience and there are rainforests to explore.

But the country's number-one attraction is the active Arenal volcano, which often puts on a fire show for tourists. On the lake at the volcano's foot, visitors can find one of Costa Rica's best windsurf spots, because winds on the lake can reach 72 kilometres per hour (45 miles per hour).

It might not be advisable to go white-water rafting after a surgical operation but that, too, is now a major attraction in the country.

FARES

Fares to San José from London start from around £500 return in economy class, with a wide choice of airlines including KLM and Delta as well as the Dutch charter Martinair.

Cosmetic surgery (and cosmetic or restorative dentistry) is Costa Rica's hidden treasure, but not a well-kept secret. In fact, a survey conducted by the University of Costa Rica as long ago as 1991 found that 14.25 per cent of all visitors to Costa Rica come to receive some sort of medical care – most often cosmetic surgery and dental work.

CROATIA

OFFICIAL NAME: Republic of Croatia
AREA: 56,610 square kilometres (21,857 square miles)
POPULATION: 4,784,265
LANGUAGE: Croatian
CAPITAL: Zagreb
TIME ZONE: Central European Time (GMT +1)
DISTANCE: London to Zagreb = 1,593 kilometres (990 miles)

Croatia has emerged from the turmoil of war in the Balkans quicker than any other region in the area, and is fast re-establishing itself as a firm favourite with tourists. Now you can combine a cultural and restful holiday in the picturesque Istrian town of Rovinj in Croatia with having all your dental work done, thanks to the modern surgery of Dr Zeljko Popadic. The clinic is well known in neighbouring countries like Hungary and Slovenia. In fact, the clinic is so highly regarded that when people think of Rovinj they automatically associate it with:

THE CLINIC FOR ESTHETIC AND IMPLANT DENTISTRY
(http://www.dr-popadic-dentist.com)
M Benussi 5, 52210 Rovinj, Croatia
Tel/Fax: +385 52 830 830
Email: dr.popadic@pu.htnet.hr

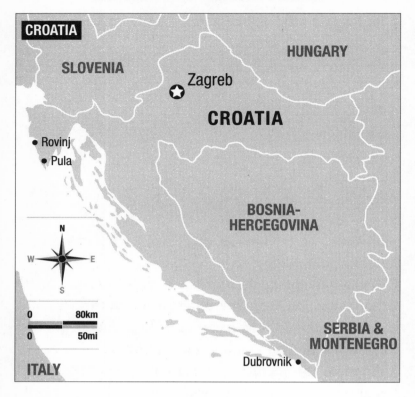

Dr. Popadic has a team that consists of two dentists, two assistants, two technicians and an administrator. It has a state-of-the-art surgery equipped with up-to-date technology and is a favourite of Austrian and Italian clients.

The clinic's price list includes:
First dental examination: €30 (£20)
Simple tooth extraction: €35 (£24)
Composite filling – one surface: €35 (£24)
Root canal treatment – incisor, canine, lower premolar: €50 (£34)

Root canal treatment – molar with 4 canals:
  €200 (£134)
Apicectomy – including apex sealing and bone grafting:
  €400 (£268)
Wisdom-tooth extraction with
alveolotomy: €200 (£134)
Gingivectomy or gingivoplasty per
quadrant: €300 (£200)
Osseous and mucogingival surgery per quadrant:
  €350 (£234)
Sinus floor elevation with bone grafting: €950 (£634)
Periodontal scaling, root planning per
  quadrant: €140 (£94)
Tartar removal – light scaling – both arches: €70 (£47)
Teeth bleaching per both arches – 5-day session:
  €250 (£167)
Complete denture – upper or lower: €580 (£387)
Immediate denture (eg after implants
  insertion): €350 (£234)
Metal-based partial with attachments
  (no clasps): €1,100 (£734)
Porcelain tooth crown or bridge element: €340 (£227)
  Veneer: €400 (£267)
Porcelain crown on implant: €355 (£237)
Procera crown (computer-designed zirconium/porcelain
  crown): €410 (£274)
Implant (Nobel Biocare, Astra Tech) and abutment:
  €1,100 (£734)
Mini implant MDL and abutment: €500 (£334)

Overdenture (attached on two implants) with bar or ball
    attachment: € 1,200 (£800)
'All-On-4' – surgical/prosthetic method including
    insertion of 4 implants and fixed acrylic bridge –
    all done in 6–8 hours, upper or
    lower: € 5,000 (£3,334)

What do Robert de Niro, Sharon Stone and Clint Eastwood have in common? They are all rumoured to be buying or have bought their own island off the coast of Croatia, and with more than 1,000 islands there are still plenty to go round. It is claimed Croatia is the new Mediterranean jewel with Istria (the area surrounding Rovinj) the new Tuscany. While staying in Rovinj you can take a day trip to Venice.

Rovinj was ruled over by the Venetian Empire for more than 500 years and its influence is still evident in the steep streets that twist around the old church of St Euphemia. The clear water bay around the town is excellent for snorkelling, and the resort of Porec and city of Pula are nearby. But don't expect Tunisian-style, white sandy beaches in Croatia; the beaches tend to be narrow and pebbly – although 58 of them fly blue flags.

Croatia is steeped in history, from the medieval cobbled streets of Rovinj to the incredible city walls of Dubrovnik, which were built between the 13th and 16th centuries. They are 82 feet high with 16 towers.

The best time to visit Croatia is between May and September, with big crowds in July and August, but warm sea for swimming until the end of September. Many leading British tour operators, such as Thomson, include not only Croatia and its more famous resorts like Dubrovnik and Porec in their brochure; they also feature Rovinj. Thomson, for instance, use four hotels in the town including two four-star. Prices including half-board and flight from the UK can be as low as £300 for seven nights, depending on when you go. If you decide to have your dental work done in the winter, then a package holiday deal makes even more sense.

FARES

Flights from London to Pula begin at around £230 for schedule airlines in economy class and £130 for charters. Schedule return flights to the capital Zagreb are from around £200 with Croatia Airlines or Malev Hungarian.

Tick-borne encephalitis, a disease preventable with a three-shot vaccination series, is found throughout inland Croatia but is not prevalent along the coast. Travellers to Croatia may obtain a list of English-speaking physicians and dentists at the American Embassy's website: www.usembassy.hr or Tel: +385 (1) 661 2376.

CYPRUS

OFFICIAL NAME: Republic of Cyprus

AREA: 9,250 square kilometres (3,571 square miles), of which 3,355 square kilometres (1,295 square miles) are in north Cyprus

POPULATION: 780,133

LANGUAGE: Greek, Turkish, English

CAPITAL: Nicosia

TIME ZONE: Three hours ahead of Greenwich Mean Time (GMT +3)

DISTANCE: London to Larnaca = 3,277 kilometres (2,036 miles)

The people speak English and drive on the left-hand side of the road, so no wonder Cyprus has been a favourite destination for British holidaymakers for years. But now, because of its modern hospitals, this developed Mediterranean island is also becoming a medical-tourist destination all year round thanks to its average of 330 days of sunshine.

Medical-tourist providers have still to discover the island in the way they have discovered European countries like Belgium, Germany and France. But one provider who has is:

THE ROYAL ARTEMIS MEDICAL CENTER
(www.hemodialysiscenter.com/home_eng.htm)

Pavlou Crineou Str, Pafos, Cyprus
Tel: +357 2696 1600 Fax +357 2696 3670
Email: contact@hemodialysiscenter.com
Offers kidney dialysis for people holidaying on the island. Simply fill in the form on their site at least four weeks before your holiday and book your treatment. They never reuse dialysers and only accept people with a recently proven negative status for HIV, HBV and HBC.

The Royal Artemis Medical Center is in a quiet residential area of town with multilingual doctors and nurses and 54 fully equipped rooms. The facilities also include a gym, aerobics room, an indoor heated pool, a Jacuzzi, an extensive sauna, steam bath, professional beautician and diet consultant. These are available to patients and their families.

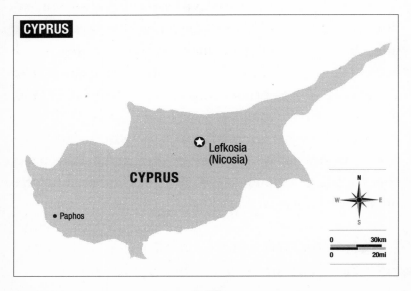

CYPRUS

The Hemodialysis Unit is equipped with Fresenius 4008S dialysis machines with the possibility of single needle. Filters are never reused. Water purification is based on reversed osmosis and dialysate on bicarbonate.

Situated off the southern coast of Turkey and the third largest island in the Mediterranean, Cyprus has good beaches, modern resorts and is riddled with Greek and Roman ruins. The country was divided in 1974 after Turks invaded and took over the northern sector. The majority of tourist development is in the south with its boisterous resorts like Ayia Napa, family areas like Larnaca and Limmosol, and Pafos, which is also a favourite with honeymooners because it is the alleged birthplace of Aphrodite, the goddess of love.

Pafos was once the capital of Cyprus in Roman and Greek time. Now it is a harbour town in the east of the country, which has spread out as tourism has embraced its beautiful setting. Its ancient sites are included in UNESCO's list of World Heritage sites and there is plenty to explore, from the Tombs of the Kings carved out of solid rock to Pafos Castle, which was originally built as a Byzantine fort. But the charming coastline, holiday amenities and surrounding mountain villages are also a major attraction for the modern visitor.

FARES
Charter flights to Pafos are available from around £120 return with scheduled airfares at £200+.

HOTELS

There are around 17,000 tourist beds in Pafos, the majority of which are pre-booked for package holidaymakers, and the high-season months of July and August see the resort packed. But worth giving a try are:

Four star: Alexander The Great (Leoforos Posidhonos, Kato Pafos, Tel: 269 65000). In an excellent position on a beach in the heart of the tourist zone. Prices C£100+.

Two star: Apollo (outskirts of Kato Pafos, Tel: 269 33909). Small and quiet with a view of the lighthouse from some rooms. Prices C£16+.

Most pharmaceutical products in Cyprus can be bought directly over the counter. There are various pharmacies on the island and many stay open late – some even for 24 hours. Non-prescription medicines are easily available and reasonably priced.

CZECH REPUBLIC

OFFICIAL NAME: Czech Republic
AREA: 78,866 square kilometres (30,450 square miles)
POPULATION: 10,241,138
LANGUAGE: Czech
CAPITAL: Prague
TIME ZONE: Two hours ahead of Greenwich Mean Time (GMT +2)
DISTANCE: London to Prague = 1,044 kilometres (649 miles)

Prague is one of the most beautiful capitals in Europe and is also a major centre for making people beautiful, thanks to the Czech Republic's strict control of cosmetic surgery.

BEAUTIFUL BEINGS
(www.beautifulbeings.co.uk/index.htm)
10 Birch Road, Stowmarket, Suffolk IP14 3EZ, UK
Tel: 0870 443 2949
Email: info@beautifulbeings.co.uk
A cosmetic-surgery agency that has chosen to focus on a clinic in Prague headed by qualified surgeon Zuzana Cerna, who worked for seven years in North America.
The clinic is within walking distance of the Old Square in Prague, and boasts top-of-the-range operating

equipment and instruments that are mostly disposable to maintain a high level of sanitation.

The prices listed include the surgery, all medications, overnight stays in a private room in the clinic, private duty nurses, all post-operative treatments and doctors' visits, the average flight cost from the UK and the appropriate accommodation for each surgical procedure. The company says that once you have been given an exact quote there are no hidden extras.

The procedures include:
Eyelid surgery (upper or lower): £1,207
Ear surgery: £1,207
Face and neck lift: £2,506
Nose surgery: £2,338
Breast enlargement and augmentation (with implant): £2,897
Breast reduction and uplift: £2,863
Tummy tuck: £2,718
Liposuction (one area): £1,957
Varicose surgery: £1,887
Hair replacement: £1,887
The company can also arrange for an independent financial organisation to help spread the cost of treatment over several years.

Accommodation, which is split into two sections so that two clients can share at any one time, can be in an apartment in Prague about 30 minutes' walk from the

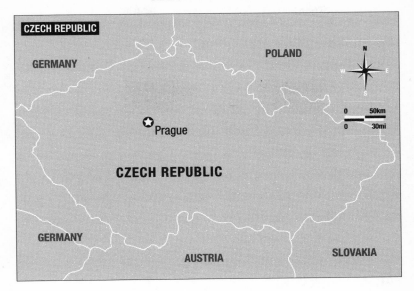

CZECH REPUBLIC

GERMANY

POLAND

Prague

CZECH REPUBLIC

GERMANY

AUSTRIA

SLOVAKIA

0   50km
0   30mi

clinic. There is also a similar apartment only five minutes' walk from the clinic. If the apartments are already booked then your accommodation can be in the FlatHotel Orion, a five-minute ride from the centre of Prague, for the same price.

Medieval towers and hundreds of church spires give a fairytale atmosphere to Prague and make it a beautiful and fascinating city to visit, combining Gothic, Baroque and Art Nouveau architecture. Since the country's arrival in the European Union, tourism to the Czech Republic has been booming and Prague is the place everyone heads for first. And there is a lot to see – from the Old Square with its cafés, bars and street entertainment to the Charles Bridge, which gives you the best view of Prague Castle at night. By day, the best view of the city is from the Observation Tower on the top of Petrin Hill.

The Prague Castle complex is the jewel in the crown with several museums to explore, and the famous Wenceslas Square is excellent for shopping as well as having all the usual fast-food restaurants.

Shopping in Prague is fun. Czech crystal glass is renowned all over the world and there are plenty of bargains to be had. It is the same with lace, which is made traditionally throughout the country. For other bargains, check out the second-hand shops in the Zizkov area.

FARES

Subject to availability, you can often get a return economy flight to Prague for under £100, although you may have to look at up to £150.

Ambulance response times can sometimes be slow in the Czech Republic and different ambulances are dispatched depending on the perceived severity of the patient's condition. Many ambulance companies also expect payment at the time of delivery.

EGYPT

OFFICIAL NAME: Arab Republic of Egypt
AREA: 1,001,450 square kilometres (386,662 square miles)
POPULATION: 77,505,756
LANGUAGE: Arabic
CAPITAL: Cairo
TIME ZONE: Two hours ahead of Greenwich Mean Time (GMT +2)
DISTANCE: London to Cairo = 3,531 kilometres (2,194 miles)

Egypt has more of the greatest wonders in the world than just about any other country – the Sphinx, the Great Pyramids at Giza and the Valley of the Kings, to name just a few – and it attracts tourists from all over the world to see them, as well as to enjoy the country's Red Sea coastal resorts. Cairo is also the Hollywood and Bollywood of the Arab world, where all the major Arabic films and Arabic pop singers hail from, so no wonder its industry in cosmetic surgery is thriving. And that surgery is available at prices far lower than in the West.

RS COSMETIC CLINIC
(www.rscosmeticclinic.com)
2 Tansley Road, North Wingfield, Chesterfield, Derbyshire S42 5JZ, UK
Tel: 01246 854927 or 0800 781 1861
Email: info@RSCosmeticClinic.com

Concentrates mainly on cosmetic surgery, but can arrange general and dental surgery as well in a clean, well-equipped hospital in Egypt.

The hospital with which the company has affiliation is the As Salam International Hospital. It is of an international standard with surgeons who have been trained in either Europe or the USA. A surgical coordinator from RS Cosmetic Clinic – a link person who is resident in Egypt – is on hand to visit the hospital and sort out any queries or worries.

The As Salam International Hospital is Egypt's pre-

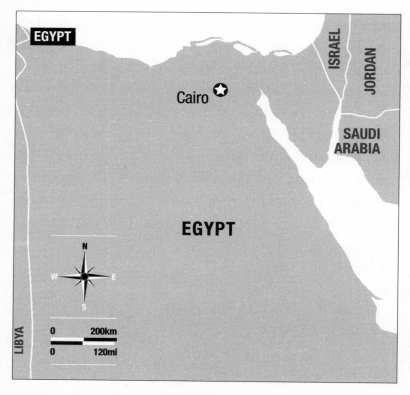

eminent major acute-care private hospital with 300 beds and is situated on the banks of the Nile looking out across the delta with views of the pyramids. All rooms have en-suite facilities.

The surgical package includes:
Pre-op surgical consultation
Pre-assessment by anaesthetist
Routine surgical procedure
Overnight stay in hospital if required
Prosthetics if required
A clinic nurse specialist with on-call telephone service
Hospital accommodation for a companion if overnight stay required.

Costs for the procedures only are:
Breast augmentation: £1,980 (€2,874)
Male gynaecomastia: £1,980 (€2,874)
Breast reduction: £2,200 (€3,194)
Breast lift: £2,200 (€3,194)
Breast lift with implants: £2,530 (€3,673)
Facelift: £1,958 (€2,843)
Blepharoplasty – upper and lower: £1,000 (€1,490)
Liposuction – one area: £1,375 (€1,995)
Liposuction – three areas: £1,595 (€2,793)
Abdominoplasty: £1,870 (€2,713)
Rhinoplasty: £1,670 (€2,423)
Otoplasty: £1,550 (€2,249)
Chin implant: £1,430 (€2,075)
Cheek implant: £1,595 (€2,314)

Botox: £310 (€449)

Total face chemical peel: £350 (€508)

Hair transplant – per three-hour session: £770 (€1,117)

Hair transplant – per six-hour session: £1,320 (€1,916)

For other procedures, contact the company.

DENTAL

One hour bleaching: £300 (€435)

EYE

Laser surgery per eye, from: £350 (€510)

The tourism package depends on the kind of holiday you want and how many people will be travelling. The company can arrange a package for two people sharing from £950 each, which will include return air travel plus 14 nights' accommodation in a five-star hotel, such as The Marriott or Hilton in Cairo, and all transfers. RS Cosmetic Clinic can also help you pick up bargain travel offers available on the Internet.

Cairo is the largest city in Africa and is teeming with millions of people. It's vibrant, electric and alive. But don't let it daunt you. The capital also offers fabulous five-star hotels that are oases of peace and calm with big swimming pools and landscaped gardens.

But no trip to Cairo, for whatever reason, is worth doing unless you take a visit to the awesome pyramids at Giza, an area that is, in fact, now a mere suburb of the great city. Visits to the pyramids, and to the spectacular sound and light show in the evenings, can be arranged by the hotel. You can travel by private air-conditioned taxi, which is strongly advised if you are recuperating from surgery, rather than battling the public transport system.

Perhaps even more worthwhile is a complete day-tour of the city, taking in not only the pyramids and sphinx at Giza but also the museum – the best antiquities museum in the world – plus the Khan el-Khalili bazaars, Islamic Cairo, with its maze of thoroughfares, and the Citadel.

If Cairo seems too much of a bustle for your recuperation, you can always take a cruise down the Nile from Luxor to Aswan in Upper Egypt. Another alternative is to relax at one of the very modern Red Sea resorts the country has to offer, such as Sharm el Sheikh, Hurghada or the newer places of Taba and Marsa Alam.

Except for during the winter months in Cairo and Alexandria, Egypt is very hot all year round and appropriate precautions against dehydration and sunburn must be taken.

Sekhmet Nefjert was the Ancient Egyptians' goddess of healing. In those times, medicine was incredibly advanced, although their cure for a headache was not quite as simple as taking paracetamol. Ancient Egyptians used to get rid of the pain by frying the skull of a catfish in oil and rubbing it on the head.

FRANCE

OFFICIAL NAME: French Republic
AREA: 547,030 square kilometres (211,210 square miles)
POPULATION: 60,656,178
LANGUAGE: French
CAPITAL: Paris
TIME ZONE: Central European Time (GMT +1)
DISTANCE: London to Paris = 346 kilometres
(215 miles)

The French health structure has always been held up as a model of modern efficiency, with no waiting system and top-notch hospitals with excellent food. The French people have been willing to put up with higher taxes than their British counterparts and pay health insurance to get to this state, and, while Belgium and Germany may be taking over from France as the top place for medical tourism in Europe, there is no denying the brilliance of the French medical system. Even the overstretched British NHS has sent patients to France in an effort to cut down on numbers.

People Logistics Ltd
(www.people-logistics.com/index.html)
Sywell Aerodrome, Northampton NN6 OBN, UK
Tel: 0800 587 9501
Email: info@people-logistics.com

Specialise in arranging all joint-replacement surgery as well as other procedures for people who are stuck on Britain's long NHS waiting lists.

They arrange a weekly service to Clinique St Isabelle,

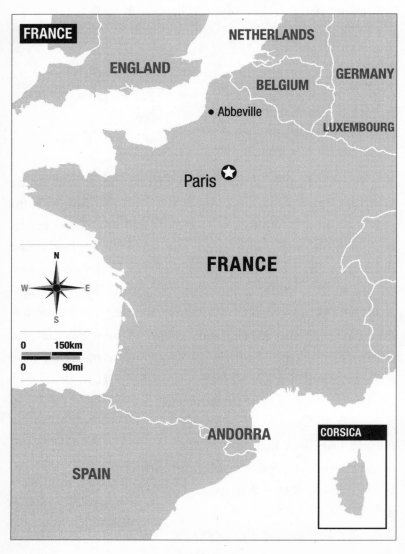

an hour south by road from Calais in the town of Abbeville. Each patient has his or her own private, en-suite room with telephone and television. The company claims the 14-day stay with a partner or companion will leave the patient fully recovered, with just the temporary use of a walking stick if necessary. The package they organise includes the 14-day stay, surgery costs, double room and all meals, hospital transfers and administration, fully escorted journey, and pre- and post-operative consultations. Prices include:

Single hip replacement: £6,350 (£6,800 including companion)

Single knee replacement: £6,850 (£7,300 including companion)

The transport used is a Mercedes V Class people carrier and the trip to France and back is through the Channel Tunnel.

In May 1940, German air raids destroyed the wooden-framed buildings that made up the town of Abbeville, so today the majority of the buildings are post-war. But there are still a few gems left, including the Collegiale St-Vulfran which was built between the 15th and 17th centuries and has been undergoing restoration ever since the war. There is also a museum overlooking the Place de l'Amiral-Courbet with paintings dating from the 16th century onwards.

Total health expenditure per person in France in 2001 was $2,567 (£1,426), which worked out at 9.6 per cent of the Gross Domestic Product. At the same time in the UK, it was only 7.5 per cent of the GDP.

GERMANY

OFFICIAL NAME: Federal Republic of Germany
AREA: 357,021 square kilometres (137,847 square miles)
POPULATION: 82,431,390
LANGUAGE: German
CAPITAL: Berlin
TIME ZONE: Central European Time (GMT +1)
DISTANCES: London to Frankfurt = 653 kilometres (406 miles)
London to Hamburg = 745 kilometres (463 miles)
London to Berlin = 946 kilometres (588 miles)
London to Munich = 940 kilometres (584 miles)

Although the German economy has been stagnating for some time, the country still boasts some of the finest medical facilities in Europe, and at prices competitive with its neighbours, Belgium and France.

And in a very smart move, a medical-tourist centre has been set up at Munich Airport so patients can fly straight in, and after treatment fly straight home again, without even having to leave the airport complex.

THE MUNICH AIRPORT CLINIC
(www.airportclinic-m.de)
Terminalstrasse West, Terminal 1, Modul E, Ebene 03,
D-85356 München-Flughafen, Germany
Tel: +49 89 975 63 328
Email: info@airportclinic-m.de

The clinic has two surgery theatres and 13 rooms. Individually designed packages can include diagnosis, inpatient or outpatient surgery, hotel accommodation, transfer to a partner clinic for long-term treatments, and

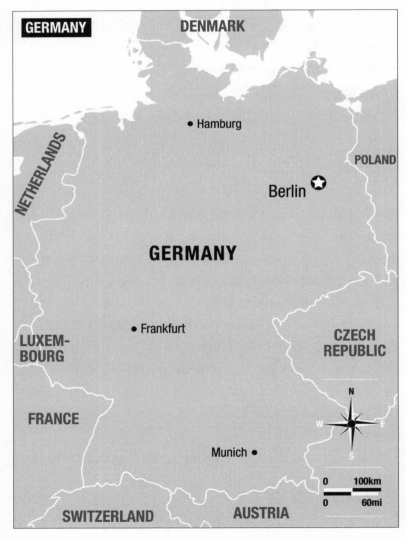

sightseeing programmes for patients and their families. The clinic will even collect patients at the aircraft and take them through immigration.

Specialities include orthopaedics, hand surgery, plastic surgery, endocrine surgery, minimally invasive surgery for various conditions, ophthalmics, ear-nose-throat medicine, urology, gynaecology, gastroenterology and treatment of cardiovascular conditions. The clinic even has a magnetic resonance imaging (MRI) scanner on the premises.

SURGICAL EXPERTS INTERNATIONAL
(www.surgicalexperts.de)
Harderstrasse 11, 85049 Ingolstadt, Germany
Tel: +49 173 8846 046 Fax: +49 841 9712 034
Email: info@surgicalexperts.de
Essentially a patient treatment-and-transfer service provider using university hospitals, community hospitals and private clinics in Germany.

They use a chauffeured service in Mercedes, BMW and Audi cars to ferry people from airports to clinics, help with hospital admission procedures and guide the patient through the hospital. They also arrange a very wide range of medical procedures with top surgeons and, although it is advised to visit the website and fill in a cost estimate for specific treatments, special offers at the time of writing include the following:

Robotic-assisted gastric bypass: €15,795 (£10,530)

This includes all consultation and medical services,

chauffeured airport pickup and ground transport, six nights in a four-star Munich hotel, return economy-class air travel, translator services, sightseeing tour and all taxes.

Conventional gastric bypass: €10,895 (£7,264)

This includes a five- to six-day hospital stay, one night's four-star hotel stay, hospital costs and taxes.

Knee-replacement packages are being offered in a hotel clinic in Bavaria with five-star service, spa and pools, luxury rooms, PGA golf course, tennis and other sports activities aimed at international patients and sports professionals.

As well as filling in the patient request form, the company also asks for your complete medical history and reports with your X-ray and ultrasound pictures, CT-scans and MRI film. This allows them to give you a better quote on costs.

GERMAN MEDICINE NET

(www.germanmedicine.net/en/)
GmbH, Yorckstrasse 23, D-79110 Freiburg
Tel: +49 761 888 730 Fax: +49 761 888 7316

The list of surgery that can be arranged through German Medicine Net is extensive, ranging from dental work to heart surgery and cosmetic treatments, and their website is very comprehensive. There is an online contact form.

The prices they quote are 'starting from' and do not include travel, hotels or the cost of hiring a translator.

But it does include their organisational fees for finding the right hospital and the right surgical team.

Here is a selection of current costs for some of the most popular procedures:

DENTAL

Standard implants (rough estimate of total costs): from €2,500 (£1,667)

Rebuilding of bone per implant: from €375 (£250)

Sinus lifting per side of face: from €1,250 (£834)

Implant: from €1,250 (£834)

Crown on implant: from €1,000 (£667)

Veneer: from €500 (£334)

ORTHOPAEDIC

Knee revision surgery: €12,500 (£8,334)

Partial knee replacement: €7,200 (£4,800)

Hip revision surgery: €12,000 (£8,000)

Hip resurfacing: €9,000 (£6,000)

CARDIAC

Bypass surgery: €11,600 (£7,734)

Mitral valve surgery: €16,000 (£10,667)

Aortic valve surgery: €14,800 (£9,867)

Stent insertion: €6,000 (£4,000)

Angiogram: €2,300 (£1,534) – partially refunded if operation follows

Balloon dilation: €1,225 (£817)

COSMETIC

Every type of cosmetic procedure can be arranged and prices can be found at:

http://geranmedicine.net/en/priceplastic.html

Here are just a few sample costs:

Liposuction (lower abdomen): €2,000 (£1,334) – 1- to 2-night stay

Botox injections: from €300 (£200)

Breast augmentation: €4,600 (£3,067) – 2- to 4-night stay

Tummy tuck: €3,500 (£2,334)

Neck lift: €1,200–1,500 (£800–1,000) – 2-night stay

Germany has some magnificent cities to visit. The capital, Berlin, is a cultural delight with three opera houses, two concert halls and eight symphony orchestras – more than any other city in the world.

Hamburg – and who hasn't heard of the famous Reeperbahn? – is an amazing city with a large lake in the middle of town, and recreational and entertainment facilities to cater for every taste.

Frankfurt, the birthplace of Goethe, is home to more than 40 museums and the seat of the Central European Bank.

Munich, with its world-famous Oktoberfest beer festival, also has magnificent architecture, more excellent museums and the lure of the Alps near by.

Apart from the elegant big cities, Germany also boasts small picture-postcard towns, castles, vineyards and, of course, the magnificent Rhine River. Germany can be visited all year round but the summer months of May to September see the greatest number of tourists.

GERMANY

Hotels and lodging are available in even the smallest of towns; prices range from €200+ (£134+) per day for a five-star hotel down to €30 (£20) for basic accommodation.

FARES

Return flights to Berlin can be as low as £50, but bank on paying £120+ if you go by schedule economy. To Hamburg, expect to pay around £100; to Frankfurt and Munich, it will cost £100+.

Almost everyone living in Germany has health insurance. Some 88 per cent belong to a statutory health scheme and around nine per cent are privately insured. Up to a certain level of income (in 2005, €3,900 gross per month or €46,800 per annum), all employees are obliged to join one of more than 315 statutory health-insurance schemes. Those earning a higher gross amount than this are free to join a private scheme if they so desire.

GREECE

OFFICIAL NAME: Hellenic Republic
AREA: 131,940 square kilometres (50,942 square miles)
POPULATION: 10,668,354
LANGUAGE: Greek
CAPITAL: Athens
TIME ZONE: Eastern European Time (GMT +2)
DISTANCE: London to Athens = 2,414 kilometres
(1,500 miles)

If you fancy looking like a Greek goddess – or a Greek god, come to that – then there is only one place to go and get your body sculptured. Greece needs no introduction to holidaymakers and is one of the most popular tourist destinations in Western Europe. And, since its highly successful staging of the Olympic Games in 2004, the popularity of this Mediterranean country, with its beautiful islands and beaches, has continued to soar.

Pilgrims and patients have been going to Greece as medical tourists since ancient times because of the healing God Asklepios at Epidaurus. With its many natural spa centres, especially those at Heraklion and Hersonissos on the island of Crete, modern Greece has an enviable reputation for thalassotherapy (therapy using seawater and sea products).

Now cosmetic surgery is available in the capital city of Athens, and the treatment can be combined with a holiday through the doctor's partner consolidators in Birmingham, UK.

Dr Nodas Kapositas
(www.kapositas.gr/en/uk.htm)
17 Dim Soutsou, Mavili Sq, Athens, Greece
Tel: +30 210 64 01 004
An international member of the American Society for Aesthetic Plastic Surgery.

Anyone from the UK seeking cosmetic treatment should contact:
Professional Capital Services
1 Victoria Square, Birmingham B1 1BD, UK
Tel: 0121 632 2000
Email: info@professionalcapital.co.uk
They can arrange bespoke travel/accommodation packages to suit personal needs.

Prices will obviously vary depending on the time of year you are planning to visit Athens and the type of accommodation required. Tours in Athens and island excursions are arranged at no extra cost after the operation.

In order to get an estimate of the cost of your medical procedure, including travel and accommodation, you'll need to fill in the enquiry form found on the website. On arrival at Athens Airport, you'll be met by a private chauffeur and driven to your hotel. The chauffeur will

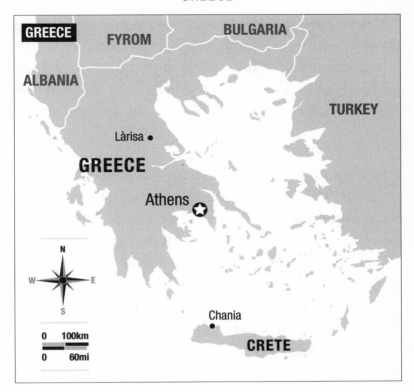

also drive you between your hotel and the clinic of Dr
Kapositas for both consultation and surgery.

Certain hotels are recommended because they are
near the medical facilities. These include the five-star
Divani Appollon Palace and Spa (www.divanis.gr) at 10
Ag Nikolaou & Iliou Str, 166 71 Athens-Vouliagmeni,
as well as the five-star Athens Hilton (www.hilton.com)
at 46 Vas. Sofias. For people on a stricter budget
there are four-star hotels as well as the three-star
Best Western Ilisia Hotel (www.bestwestern.com) at
25 Michalakopoulou Str.

Depending on your operation and its healing process, you may be able to take advantage of a free one-day tour of Athens, an island excursion to Aigina, Spetses, Poros and Hydra, or even the cosmopolitan Mykonos and Santorini, during the spring-summer period.

Other Greek medical-tourist providers are becoming available, and one is actively co-operating with **The Vardinoyannion Eye Institute of Crete** (www.greek-holidays.net/medical/), which offers many procedures including laser techniques for cataracts, cornea and retina work and transplantation.

The University Hospital of Larissa
Mezourio, Greece
Tel: +30 24 10 6 82 795
Has an Assisted Reproduction Unit which provides IVF, ICSI and intrauterine insemination as well as storage for embryos, eggs and sperm.

The Fertility Center Chania
(www.fertilitycenter-crete.gr/)
Markou-Botsary 64A, Chania 73136, Crete, Greece
Tel: +30 69 722 47 074 Fax: +30 28 210 76 106
Email: info@fertilitycenter-crete.gr
Offers holiday packages that can be organised through the liaison manager. The procedures include IVF and ICSI as well as Assisted Hatching (AH) and Blastocyst

embryo development. The hotels used all boast five-star-style facilities.

Initial contact with the centre should be made by email, phone or fax in order to set up a consultation with gynaecologist Dr Ioannis Giakoumakis. The website gives a very comprehensive step-by-step IVF cycle timeline, from the early down-regulation of the ovaries to the final procedures and holiday in Crete.

FARES
EasyJet fly from both Luton and Gatwick to Athens with fares depending on how far in advance you book, but you should be looking at less than £100 return. The city is also catered for by many scheduled services, which can be as low as £150. Bucket shops offer good deals on flights to Chania in Crete, with charters as low as £100 and schedules up to £250.

Hippocrates and other Ancient Greek practitioners argued that the Four Humours – blood, phlegm, yellow bile and black bile – needed to be balanced for people to remain healthy. It resulted in doctors looking for symptoms for the first time and was the basis upon which medical reasoning developed.

HUNGARY

OFFICIAL NAME: Republic of Hungary
AREA: 93,030 square kilometres (35,919 square miles)
POPULATION: 10,006,835
LANGUAGE: Hungarian
CAPITAL: Budapest
TIME ZONE: Central European Time (GMT +1)
DISTANCE: London to Budapest = 1,485 kilometres
(923 miles)

No wonder Hungarians smile a lot! No other country has more dentists per head of population. And since the country joined the European Union their fellow Europeans have had plenty to smile about, too, because prices are considerably cheaper there than in neighbouring countries like Austria and Germany.

Now British citizens are getting in on the act thanks to a British-based company that specialises in dental medical tourism to Hungary. And another British company is offering general surgery, orthopaedic procedures and infertility treatment at a top hospital near the Hungarian capital of Budapest.

Smile Savers Hungary
(www.smilesavershungary.co.uk/)
234B Battersea Bridge Road, London, SW11 3AA, UK
Tel: 020 7585 2742

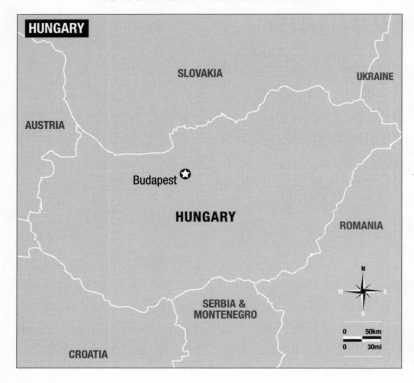

Email: customerservices@smilesavershungary.co.uk

The company specialises in finding dentists and clinics in Budapest that are suitable for UK clients. They claim that all their customers come back with the 'wow' factor thanks to the high quality of service, clinics with the latest technology, guaranteed workmanship, fair prices, and clinics that are open out-of-hours and at weekends for clients in a hurry.

Their comprehensive website allows customers to pick a dentist to suit, look around their clinic, check live flight prices, and even get a quick estimate of the total cost of the visit.

Clinics include one run by Dr Bela Batorfi in the suburbs of Budapest, which is situated above his family home and contains state-of-the-art modern dental equipment.

The Implant and Aesthetic Centre is an impressive clinic situated in the affluent hill area of Buda. One of the team dentists, Dr Attila Kaman, has placed more than 15,000 implants in the last 12 years. The clinic boasts an array of specialists and dental assistants.

Dr Renner's clinic is on the banks of the Danube close to the centre of Budapest in a modern office block. As the chief dentist and qualified medical practitioner, Dr Renner guarantees personal attention.

Here is a rough guide to the prices you can expect to pay for dental treatment in Hungary through Smile Savers:

Consultation: Free	
X-ray:	£30
Tooth whitening:	£450
Composite filling:	£50
Extraction:	£30
Root canal treatment:	£80
Porcelain veneer:	£180
Ceramic inlay:	£180
Porcelain crown:	£180
Porcelain fused to gold:	£250
Bridge units/tooth:	£180
Denture with plastic tooth/arch:	£300
Denture with ceramic tooth/arch:	£600
Gnathological treatment:	£215
Implant:	£580

For a more accurate quotation of treatment, Smile Savers Hungary need an X-ray to be sent to them. The quotation can be given within three days while the patient is in the UK.

PERFECT PROFILES
(http://www.perfectprofiles.eu.com/)
30 Bedford Road, Houghton Regis,
Bedfordshire LU5 5DJ, UK
Tel: 0870 128 0636 Fax: 0870 128 0636
Email: enquiries@perfectprofiles.eu.com
Offers the opportunity to have surgical and medical treatments at the first private hospital in Hungary, which was set up in 1998. The Telki Hospital, near Budapest, has 100 inpatient beds. Patient rooms are of a high standard with air-conditioning, private bathroom, telephone, satellite TV, radio and Internet access. The room can be a double or single according to choice. A restaurant and café are at the service of patients in the hospital, and patients' relatives or friends can stay in the room free of charge.

The company can arrange all the usual cosmetic procedures like facelifts, breast surgery and even tattoo removal – based at a clinic in the Hotel Thermal – as well as dental, laser eye and general surgery, orthopaedic and infertility treatment. Heart check-ups can also be arranged at a unique cardiac clinic.

Accommodation can be arranged by the company. It ranges from the four-star Spa Hotel Thermal to city hotels, and staff are on hand to meet patients at the airport and also arrange all transfers.

Dental-surgery prices can be found on the Perfect Profiles website and the cost of other treatments can be obtained from the company by filling in a request form. Prices do not include flights. If you are undecided about whether you want to use the company, they can arrange pre-inspection visits with a two-night break from £99, flight cost additional.

KREATIV DENTAL TOURS
(www.kreativdent.co.uk/)
25 Uplands Road, Rumney, Cardiff CF3 3AN, UK
Tel: 0292 031 2608 Fax: 0870 130 1975
This company claims it is driven by quality and not the lowest prices, and relies solely on one surgery in Budapest established in May 1996. It consists of a fully equipped surgery combined with an advanced laboratory. Four internationally experienced dentists work in the dental surgery with three hygienists, supported by a dental laboratory with six technicians, all of whom speak English. The company advises that a one-week visit is normally more than enough for most crown and bridge work, and implants require a 10- to 12-day stay with a return visit of 6 days after about 4–6 months.

They like at least two weeks' notice of anyone wanting treatment so they can have time to organise appointments, accommodation and flights. The company has featured in many of Britain's top newspapers, including the *Sunday Times*, the *Daily Telegraph* and the *Sun*, as well as appearing on the BBC. Here is an example of their prices, which may fluctuate and change:

Consultation: Free
Dental hygienic treatment: £60
Conventional tooth whitening upper/lower (bleaching kit and foil last for 8 days, patient does it her/himself): £150
BriteSmile/Remewhite Tooth Whitening System upper/lower treatment, performed during 1 session (one-and-a-half-hours long, done by dentist): £280

Extraction:	£32
Root canal treatment/canal:	£65
Composite filling:	£68
GC GRADIA ceramic/composite inlay:	£160
Post/core:	£50
Porcelain crown fused to metal (gold extra):	£180
Porcelain fused to 24k Galvan gold (gold included):	£250
Aesthetic shoulder porcelain:	£33
GC GRADIA full porcelain/composite crown:	£230
Full cast metal crown:	£130.00
Temporary crown:	Free
GC GRADIA veneer:	£180.00
Denture upper or lower (complete with teeth):	£330
Telescopic crown (primary and secondary):	£220
Denture reline/rebase:	£46

Gnathological treatment:	£285
Implant:	£580
Gold surcharge:	£68

Kreativ Dental Tours arranges accommodation at the Hotel Amadeus, which is five minutes away from the dental facility and 15 minutes from the city centre. The hotel, built in 1992, has 39 rooms with bath, phone and satellite TV and a special menu is provided for patients of Kreativ Dental. It is offered at a discounted price of around £30 per night for a double room with breakfast, and £20 for a single (prices at the time of writing).

Clients are also encouraged to use low-cost carriers such as SkyEurope from Stansted to Budapest, or Easyjet from Luton, and the company provides free transport to and from the airport by private car. They also welcome package tourists who happen to be in Budapest and fancy dental surgery.

DR VOLOM AESTHETIC AND GENERAL DENTAL SURGERY
(http://www.dreamsmile.hu/)
1011 Budapest, Fö utca 37/c
Tel: +36 30 520 2000 Fax: +36 14 89 3709
Email: info@dreamsmile.hu
Dr Volom offers a guarantee that, if your dental work fails and you must have repair work done in the UK, then you can forward the bill to him, or you can return to Budapest where treatment will be free and he will pay the travel and hotel bills. The surgery offers a wide

range of dental treatments including a free consultation and X-ray.

Here are just a few of the prices for treatment. The full range can be found on the website:

Tooth bleaching (one-and-a-half hours in office):	£400
Root canal (1 root):	£80
Two roots:	£100
Three roots:	£134
Porcelain veneer or inlay:	£148
Full porcelain jacket crown:	£220
Swedish implants per piece:	£650
Plastic and metal combination dentures:	£400

The practice recommends using the NH Hotel Budapest for accommodation because it is located near the office and offers a discount price of €78 (£52) a night if booked through them.

BEAUTY HUNGARY

(http://www.beautyhungary.com/)
Email: info@beautyhungary.com
This is a new operation based in Budapest offering to integrate health, beauty, travel and leisure. They prepare tailor-made package deals for people wanting cosmetic or dental surgery. The website was still under construction at the time of writing.

Prices for dentistry are competitive:

Porcelain veneer:	£160

Implant:	£600
Teeth whitening:	£300

Budapest is famous for its Turkish baths, which is not surprising considering there is no other capital city in the world with nearly 100 thermal springs and 12 medicinal baths within its boundaries, where 19 million gallons of thermal water rise to the surface each day.

The city straddles the River Danube and has broad avenues and green parks with a turn-of-the-century feel that exudes elegance. Its attractions are many, from the opulence of the 1884 opera house with its breathtaking interior, to its number-one tourist destination – Castle Hill – with its monuments, museums and great views across the Danube to Pest. The Old Town is particularly enthralling, with its medieval streets and striking painted houses.

The bath houses are, of course, not to be missed, particularly the Kiraly on Fö utca. The baths are clean, cheap and safe, but remember they tend to become a gay venue on male-only days.

FARES
Thanks to budget airlines like EasyJet and Wizz, you can fly to Budapest for as little as £17 one-way depending on how far in advance you book. Schedule flights are also available, with prices from £90 to £140 return.

The mofette (a vent in the Earth's crust) in Mátraderecske, northern Hungary, is a truly unusual feature in the field of medical science. This so-called dry bath employs naturally occurring carbon dioxide of volcanic origin and is recommended for the treatment of heart conditions and circulatory disorders, blood pressure irregularities and dermatological complaints.

INDIA

OFFICIAL NAME: Republic of India
AREA: 3,287,590 square kilometres (1,269,346 square miles)
POPULATION: 1,080,264,388
LANGUAGE: Hindi is the national language and there are 14 other official languages
CAPITAL: New Delhi
TIME ZONE: India Time (GMT +5.5)
DISTANCES: London to Mumbai (Bombay) = 7,207 kilometres (4,478 miles)
London to Delhi = 6,727 kilometres (4,180 miles)
London to Calcutta = 7,979 kilometres (4,958)
London to Chennai (Madras) = 8,228 kilometres (5,113 miles)
London to Colombo, Sri Lanka = 8,708 kilometres (5,411 miles)

If one country can claim the crown as the world centre for medical tourism, it has to be India. The same far-sightedness that has seen this impoverished country rise to become one of the world's great economic powerhouses, along with China, in the last 10 years has also set it on the road to capturing the growing army of worldwide medical tourists.

Brand-new state-of-the art hospitals, which Britain's NHS can only dream about, have been built in the main cities of the subcontinent. Theatre apparatus usually consists of the very latest German and Danish products. And, with its cheap labour force of skilled professional doctors and ancillary workers, treatment costs have been driven down to highly accessible levels.

The medical-tourism industry has also been given a fillip by the Indian government, which has declared it an

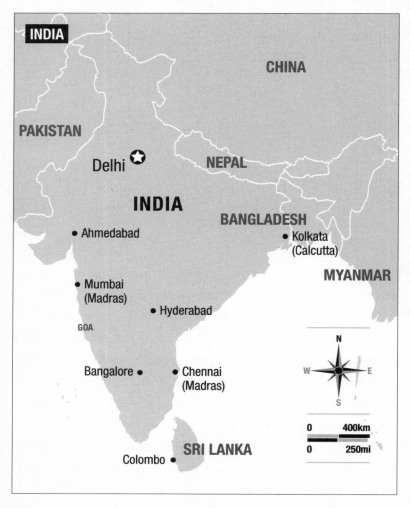

export industry with all the tax breaks and incentives that that implies.

And now Thomas Cook is expected to test the market with 'sun and surgery' package deals to India that include flights, operations, accommodation and restful recuperation. The number of British patients seeking treatment in India is expected to rise to several thousand a year, swelling the 150,000 international health visitors that flocked to the country last year. And it is easy to see why, with advanced heart surgery costing £6,000 in Mumbai (Bombay) compared with £30,000 in the UK.

By the year 2012, India is expected to be earning £1 billion a year from medical tourism. One private Indian hospital group has even offered to ease the burden on Britain's 'Third World' NHS system by taking waiting-list patients and saving the UK taxpayers money. But the British government has turned down the offer, saying NHS patients are not allowed to fly for more than three hours for treatment.

APOLLO GROUP
(www.apollohospdelhi.com/apollo-group/index.html)
This is the largest healthcare company in Asia, with international hospitals in Indian cities like Hyderabad, New Delhi and Ahmedabad, as well as a speciality hospital in Chennai (Madras). The Apollo Group caters for every possible type of treatment and procedure, and everything included in Section One of this handbook –

except LASIK eye surgery – plus a lot more can be treated at an Apollo Hospital.

The price of any treatment is much cheaper, for an internationally high standard, than anywhere else in the world. Costs are worked out on a patient's needs and can include the holiday stay and accommodation, all of which can be arranged by an international liaison officer at the hospital.

As a rule of thumb, procedures cost about half what they would in Europe or about a quarter of what you would expect to pay privately in the UK. Here are some examples of the cost of a few procedures (excluding holiday stay):

Breast augmentation without implants:

$2,390 (£1,328)

Implants for breast augmentation –

per pair: $1,150 (£639)

Birmingham hip resurfacing: $6,000 (£3,334)

One cycle IVF: $2,750 (£1,528)

Whole-body check-up: $155 (£86)

INDRAPRASTHA APOLLO HOSPITAL NEW DELHI
(www.apollohospdelhi.com/index.html)
Sarita Vihar, Delhi-Mathura Road, New Delhi 110076
Tel: +91 11 2692 5801/5858 Fax: +91 11 2682 3629
Email: helpdesk_delhi@apollohospitals.com
This is the largest corporate hospital outside of the United States. It is a 695-bed hospital with the provision to expand to 1,000 beds. It provides a wide

range of services for international patients including airport pick-up and drop, local sightseeing, hotel accommodation, translators, visa assistance and food to suit your palate.

International patients should contact Ms Paulami Karnwal by phone or fax, or email her at: paulami_k@apollohospitals.com.

The hospital has a cancer and a cardiac centre as well as institutes for orthopaedics, organ transplants, dental surgery, fertility clinic and much more, together with neurosurgery. They also do health check-ups, starting from $30 (£17) for a breast check-up to $150 (£83) for a complete body check for international patients.

APOLLO HOSPITAL HYDERABAD
(http://www.apollohospitalgroup.com/the_apollo_hyd.htm)
Jubilee Hills, Hyderabad 500033
Tel: +91 40 2360 7777 Fax: +91 40 2360 8050
Email: apollohyd@apollolife.com
The second in the Apollo chain of hospitals, with a bed capacity of 600. Located in the idyllic and peaceful Jubilee Hills, it is the largest multi-speciality healthcare facility in Hyderabad. It prides itself on being the healthcare destination for the global community and boasts its own helipad. It has an International Patient Care Office, with a first-aid and help desk at the arrival terminal at Hyderabad Airport to ensure that patients and families are cared for right from the time of landing at Hyderabad.

The wellness centre at the 30-acre hospital campus offers gymnasium, yoga, meditation, pebble walk and other facilities for holistic healthcare. Guest-room facilities are available to accommodate the families of patients. The air-conditioned single-patient rooms are equipped with nurse-call systems, satellite television, refrigerator and telephone. Cuisine is international.

Patients from abroad should contact Mr Radhey Mohan or email: gmoperations@123india.com.

Once again, most medical procedures are available, but, if the Hyderabad hospital can't cater for you, they will advise you on the best Apollo Hospital to contact.

APOLLO GLENEAGLES HOSPITAL, KOLKATA
58 Canal Circular Road, Kolkata 54, West Bengal
Tel: +91 33 2358 5218/2321 1553.
The website for this 325-bed 50-speciality hospital was still under construction at the time of writing, but information can be gleaned from www.apollohospitals.com/grouphospitals/grouphospitals_more.asp?place=kol.

The hospital, in the city formerly known as Calcutta, is jointly promoted by Apollo Hospitals and the Singapore-based Parkway Group, and has become the healthcare hub not only for northeastern India but also for Bangladesh, Nepal and Myanmar. All the services you would expect from a top-line Apollo Hospital are available including:

Orthopaedics/spine surgery
Radiology
Cardiology and cardiothoracic surgery
Vascular/visceral surgery
Gastroenterology
Nephrology and urology
Oncology
Ear, nose and throat surgery
Maxillo-facial and cosmetic surgery
General surgery
Neurology and neurosurgery
Paediatrics
Respiratory medicine
Ophthalmology

APOLLO HOSPITAL AHMEDABAD
This 400-bed multi-speciality hospital was opened in May 2003 in the capital city of Mahatma Gandhi's home state. Marble temples and age-old palaces, as well as a water-themed park, are all features of the city, which makes it an excellent tourist resort. The hospital undertakes all the treatments and procedures that are available in the Kolkata establishment.

APOLLO HOSPITAL COLOMBO
(http://www.apollocolombo.com
578 Elvitigala Mawatha, Narahenpita,
Colombo 5, Sri Lanka
Tel: +94 74 539 005 Fax: +94 74 511 199

Situated in the capital of Sri Lanka, an independent island country off the southern tip of India, this hospital was opened in 2002 and is similar to the complexes in Kolkata and Ahmedabad offering more than 50 specialities.

APOLLO SPECIALITY HOSPITAL CHENNAI
(www.apollohospitals.com)
21 Greams Lane, Chennai 600 006
Tel: +91 44 2829 0200/2829 3333
Fax: +91 44 2829 4429
Email: enquiry@apollohospitals.com
This hospital offers exclusive care in super specialities such as oncology, neurology, neurosurgery, ENT, orthopaedics and cosmetic surgery. Situated in the city formerly known as Madras, it has been rated the number-one hospital in India in the private sector for the last two years. It has carried out 7,000 heart surgeries with a success rate of 99.6 per cent – on a par with global standards – a 70 per cent success rate in bone-marrow transplants, and is the first hospital in India to do total knee replacement and the latest Illizarov procedure.

Because of its private status, the hospital is aimed exclusively at international patients – for which a special office has been set up – and the growing middle class of India.

Testimonials from UK patients include a 44-year-old woman who had a knee operation and said, 'The cost of medical treatment was the final clincher, which was

£2,500 as against £10,000 for what we would have paid for in a private facility in the UK. We were informed that the treatment would take three weeks and I can say without a doubt that this has been the best three weeks of my life.'

A 29-year-old man from South Wales, who had a Birmingham Hip Replacement (resurfacing), spent 11 days at the hospital in an air-conditioned en-suite room with all treatment and meals, said, 'Should I tell you the price? All expenses including new passport, visas, two return tickets, ambulance to airport for return journey, cardiac check-up, all for less than £5,000. Only wished I had done it years back, I would have saved myself untold agony.'

A gap of seven to ten days is advised after discharge from hospital before taking a long-haul international flight. The hospital has negotiated a special price for patients in two of the seaside resorts close to Chennai.

THE TEMPLE BAY BEACH RESORT

(www.nivalink.com/templebay) is a five-star property with 72 deluxe cottages fully equipped with air-conditioning and colour satellite TVs. There is a restaurant, swimming pool and landscaped gardens. Prices cost from £43 (€65) a day for a chalet single, to £77 (€115) for a villa double with sea view. Local taxes are extra, but the hospital can get a discount.

The five-star beach resort of **Fisherman's Cove** (www.tajhotels.com/Leisure/Fishermans%20Cove,CHE

NNAI/default.htm) at Covelong Beach, Kanchipuram District 603 11 is run by the Taj Hotel Group, has 88 cottages and can be booked online.

THE TAJ MEDICAL GROUP
(http://www.tajmedicalgroup.co.uk/index.html)
The Gallery, 275 Cromwell Lane, Kenilworth, Warwickshire CV8 1PN, UK
Tel: 0800 1076 360
Email: info@tajmedicalgroup.co.uk
The Taj Medical Group is a British-based company that specialises in knee and hip replacement, cardiac, prostate, cataract, cosmetic, dental and neurosurgery, and comprehensive preventative healthcare checks at top-rated hospitals in India.

The costs of procedures that can be arranged by the Group include all theatre, surgeon and anaesthetist's costs, nursing and medical care, drugs and dressings and private accommodation.

Examples of prices include:
Cardiac bypass: £6,400
Hip replacement: £2,600
Knee replacement: £2,400
Cataract removal: £650
MRI Scan: £120
Liposuction/tummy tuck: £800–1,200
Rhinoplasty: £900–1,500
Hysterectomy: £800–1,000

The company can arrange for treatment in the holiday resort of Goa as well as the upmarket medical shopping mall of Health City in Bangalore, where there are separate hospitals for orthopaedic surgery, cosmetic surgery and cardiac procedures.

The Taj Medical Group boasts an extensive knowledge of privately owned hospitals and specialist clinics throughout India comprising more than 250 specialist doctors, dentists, surgeons and anaesthetists as part of The Taj Medical Group Limited.

Averill Dollery from Worcestershire was barely able to walk because of the pain in her back from a pinched spinal cord, and yet for 13 years she was on Britain's National Health Service waiting list.

'It was always, ' "Just go away and take your tablets",' says Averill. 'I was told by British doctors that spinal surgery was too risky because of my weight problem.'

Things got worse until Averill decided she had to do something about the chronic pain, which was now also affecting her knee. With the help of The Taj Medical Group, she elected to go to India for an operation at the Apollo Hospital in New Delhi. The operation cost one third of what it would have cost in a private hospital in the UK.

The procedure to fuse Averill's spine took nearly three hours; it was a success, and the surgeon also decided to carry out a knee replacement. Two weeks after the operation Averill took her first steps, and a few days later she was preparing to leave India with her husband, Roger, who had accompanied her.

He says, 'India saved Averill's life. Thank you is not enough. Averill's pain was so bad, she may have felt strongly about taking her own life if it had carried on, and I would have helped her, no qualms.'

THE MEDICAL TOURIST COMPANY

(www.medicaltourist.co.uk)
PO Box 467, Harrow, Middlesex HA2 2AX, UK
Tel: 0845 838 2291 Fax: 0845 838 1325
Email: info@medicaltourist.co.uk
This is a UK-based company that offers a complete service package from arranging treatment, travel, concierge services, accommodation and visas to contacting the hospitals and doctors directly. Their main destination is India and Dr Premhar Shah, who has been practising medicine for more than 30 years, heads the company. Their prices include transfers to and from the hospital and accommodation for one person, but do not include flights. They can also arrange tailor-made packages.

Here are some basic costs:
Knee replacement: £5,000
Hip replacement: £4,500
Coronary artery bypass grafting: £7,500
Coronary angioplasty: £3,000
Dental implants: £600
Executive health check-up: £149

Squint correction: £700
Cataract removal: £700
LASIK (per eye): £500
Gall-bladder removal: £2,000
Haemorrhoids removal: £700

MEDICAL TOURISM INDIA
(http://www.medicaltourismindia.com/index.html)
Erco Reizen, Dordtselaan 144d 3073 GL, Rotterdam,
The Netherlands
Tel: +31 10 484 9177 Fax: +31 10 484 6534
Email: erco.reizen@wxs.nl
Medical Tourism India arranges complete packages,
which include treatment and tours of India, and has
offices both on the sub-continent and in Mauritius.
Their main treatment packages are for dental care, eye
care, heart care, heart surgery, health check-ups,
cosmetic treatment and orthopaedic surgery.

The company uses the Apollo Hospitals as well as the
Tata Memorial Hospital in Mumbai (Bombay), The
Institute for Cardiovascular Disease in Chennai (Madras)
and the Birla Heart Research Centre in Calcutta.

To any of those treatment packages you can add a
holiday package such as:

GOLDEN TRIANGLE TOUR
Destinations covered: Delhi–Agra–Jaipur–Delhi
Duration: 7 days (6 nights)

RAJASTHAN CULTURAL TOUR
Destinations covered:
Delhi–Varanasi–Agra–Fatehpur Sikri and more cities
Duration: 24 days (23 nights)

KERALA BACKWATER TOUR
Destinations covered:
Cochin–Periyar–Kumarakom–houseboat–Marari–
Cochin
Duration: 8 days (7 nights)

TAJ MAHAL AND TIGER TOUR
Destinations covered:
Delhi–Agra–Bandhavgarh–Delhi
Duration: 10 days (9 nights)

PALACE ON WHEELS TOUR
Destinations covered:
Delhi–Jaipur–Jaisalmer–Jodhpur–Sawai Madhopur
and more cities
Duration: 8 days (7 nights)
For full costs, contact the company.

MED DE TOUR
(http://www.meddetour.com/index.html)
4 Court Drive, Maidenhead, Berkshire SL6 8LX, UK
Tel: 0870 3800 516 Fax: 01628 778 244
Email: info@meddetour.com

A UK-based company with operations in India, which offers medical and health treatments ranging from open-heart surgery to liposuction combined with leisure holiday packages. One of the hospitals they use is the Manipal in Bangalore which has 650 beds and deals in more than 39 specialities. The company arranges appointments, accommodation and hospital stays in India as well as a tailor-made holiday after surgery.

Here is an example of some of their prices for different procedures:
Coronary angiogram: £180–310
Coronary angioplasty: £580–1,150
Open-heart surgery: £1,750–3,100
Circumcision: £100–200
Knee replacement: from £3,200
Hip replacement: £3,700
Cataract removal: £165–410
Hernia: £570–1,450
Hysterectomy: £520–1,350
Tonsillectomy: £125–300
Squint correction: £175–420
Eyelid surgery: £380–1,000
Nose reshaping: £560–1,370
Liposuction: £440–1,100

ESCORTS HEART INSTITUTE AND RESEARCH CENTRE
(http://www.ehirc.com)
Okhla Road, New Delhi 110 025

Tel: +91 11 2682 5000 Fax: +91 11 2682 5013
Email: contact@ehirc.com
EHIRC is dedicated to all aspects of cardiac surgery, and has a special office to streamline the arrival and stay of medical tourists. They offer visa assistance and arrange outside lodging in either a hotel or guesthouse. All travel and ticketing arrangements for both patients and relatives can be made, and clients are collected from the airport by either car or ambulance. Local travel needs for sightseeing, shopping and even prayer are undertaken, and they can exchange money. For the cost of procedures for overseas patients, there is a special email address for the marketing department: mktg@ehirc.com.

The hospital is located in south Delhi, 30 kilometres (19 miles) from the airport. It has 326 beds and nine operating theatres, and boasts state-of-the-art facilities and technologies.

Here is a list of private hospitals in India with world-class clinical facilities:

All India Heart Foundation, 4874 Ansari Nagar, 24 Dariya Ganj, New Delhi – 110002.

Apollo Heart Hospitals, 21 Greams Lane, Off Greams Road, Chennai – 600006. Tel: +91 11 8277 447/8240 200 Fax: +91 44 8324 429.

Apollo Hospitals, Jubilee Hills, Hyderabad – 500034. Tel: +91 40 238 050.

Bangalore Hospital Ltd, Vijaya Mallaya Hospital, No 2 Vittal Mallaya Road, Bangalore – 560001.

Batra Hospital and Medical Research Centre, 1 Tughlakabad Institutional Area, MB Road, New Delhi – 110062. Tel: +91 11 6983 747/6982 455.

Breach Candy Hospital and Research Centre, 60 Bhulabhai Desai Road, Mumbai – 400028.

Calcutta Imaging Institute, 54 Jawahar Lal Nehru Road, Calcutta – 700071.

CDR Groups of Hospitals, CDR Heart Institute, Hyderabad – 500029.

Chaitram Hospital and Research Centre, Manik Bagh Road, Indore – 452001.

Chandigarh Neurological Research Centre, 156–158 Sector 170C, Chandigarh.

Christian Medical College Heart Research Centre, Christian Medical College, Ludhiana – 141008. Christian Medical College Hospital, Vellore – 362004. Tel: +91 416 22102.

East Coast Hospital Ltd, 133 Hundred Feet Road, Natesan Nagar, Pondicherry.

Dayanad Medical College and Hospital, Post Box No 265, Ludhiana – 141001.

Deccan Hospitals, Deccan Hospital Corporation Ltd, 1–11–252/11/1, Begumpet, Hyderabad – 500016.

Diwan Chand Satya Pal Aggarwallmaging Research Centre, 10-B, Kasturba Gandhi Marg, New Delhi – 110001.

Down Town Hospital Pvt Ltd, Gaha Lodge, Guwahati – 781001.

Dr Balabhai Nanavati Hospital, SV Road, Vile Park (West), Mumbai – 400056.

Dr Babasaheb Ambedkar Vaidyakiya Pratishthan's Dr Hedgewar Hospital, Sindhuteer, Bhagyanagar, Aurangabad – 431001.

Guwahati Neurological Research Centre Pvt Ltd, Dispur, Guwahati, Assam – 781006.

Indian Cancer Society, Delhi Branch, B-82, Defence Colony, New Delhi – 110024.

Institute of Cardio-Vascular Diseases, 4-A, Jayalalitha Nagar, Mogappair, Chennai – 600050.
Tel: +91 44 6259 801 (10 lines)
Fax: +91 44 6259 804.

Jaslok Hospital and Research Centre, 15 Dr Go Deshmukh Marg, Mumbai – 400026.

Kasturba Medical College, Madhava Nagar, Manipal, Karnataka – 576119.

Kasturba Medical College, Manipal, Udupi Distt – 576199.

Key Pee Kay Medical Services (P) Ltd, 43 Second Main Road, Raja Annamalai Puram, Madras – 28.

Lady Willington Nursing Home, 21 Pycrofts Garden Road, Chennai – 06.

Lion's Cancer Detection Centre Trust, Govt Medical College Campus, Majura Gate, Surat – 395001.

Madras Medical Mission, Institute of CV Diseases, 180-NSK, Salai, Chennai – 26.

Manipal Hospital, 98 Rustom Bagh, Airport Road, Bangalore – 560017.

Medwin Hospitals, Jaya Diagnostic and Research Centre Ltd, 100 Raghave Ratna Towers, Chirag Ali Lane, Hyderabad – 500001.

Meenakshi Mission Hospital and RC Lake Area, Malur Road, Madurai – 01.

Meherbai Tata Memorial Hospital, Stocking Road, Jamshedpur – 8310001.

MI Diagnostic and Research Centre, B-22, Kailash Colony, New Delhi – 110048.

Nanda Hospital and Scan Research Centre Pvt Ltd, 0/63, Doctor's Coloney, Kankar Bagh, Patna – 20.

National Heart Institute, 49 Community Centre, East of Kailash, New Delhi – 65.

Navin Chand Nanda National Institute of Echo-cardiology and Cardiac Research, Mool Chand, RR Research Hospital, Lajapat Nagar–III, New Delhi – 110024.

PD Hinduja National Hospital and Medical Research Centre, Veer Sayarkar Marg, Mahim, Mumbai – 400016.

Parent's Association Thalassemic Unit Trust (Regd), St. George's Hospital, Mumbai – 400001.

Peerless Hospital and Research Centre Ltd, 360 Panchasayar, Garia, Calcutta – 84, West Bengal.

Ramachandra Educational and Health Trust, 25 Sir CV Raman Road, Alwarpet, Madras – 600018.

Ramakrishan Mission Hospital, OP RK Mission, Itanager – 791113, Arunachal Pradesh.

Sir Gangaram Hospital, Sir Gangaram Hospital Marg, New Delhi – 110060.

St John's Medical College Hospital, Sarjah Pur Road, Bangalore – 5600034.

St Stephen's Hospital, Tis Hazari, Delhi – 110054.

Suniti Devi Singhania Hospital and MRC, New Hind House, N Morarjee Marg, Ballard Estate, Mumbai – 400038.

Tamil Nadu Hospital Ltd, No 18 East Street, Kamraj Nagar, Thiruvamayur, Madras – 41.

The Heart Institute, Vijaya Health Centre, Vijaya Gardens, NSK Salai, Vadapalani, Madras – 26.

Vijay Mallaya Hospital Ltd, McDowell, No 17 Richmond Road, Bangalore – 25.

Seema Vyas from England says, 'I had been considering laser eye surgery for a few years and, after a Medical Tourism Exhibition in England, I was attracted to the idea of getting it done in India. The cost was a major factor as I could enjoy a holiday, do some shopping and get my eyes sorted out for less than it would cost me in England.

'I researched various eye hospitals, and finally decided on "Perfect Vision" because of the quality of the website, and the location in Faridabad, Haryana, India. All queries were answered promptly when I made contact by email. I was made to feel very comfortable by the staff – they were very friendly, gave clear explanations and had a professional manner. As I have been wearing glasses since I was eight years old, being able to see without the aid of glasses or contact lenses is a very big thing for me. "Perfect Vision" have certainly lived up to their name, and I'm very satisfied with the whole experience. I would like to thank all the staff and highly qualified doctors for changing my life for the better.'

Although India has the perfect combination of very low medical costs and very high-tech hospitals with highly trained doctors, it is a long-haul destination and might not be suitable for everyone. The flight to India from the UK is about nine hours, and, although the hospitals are all air-conditioned, the main cities can be stiflingly hot. Even in its cool season, Chennai can be hotter than the UK in the summer and acclimatisation is necessary before real recuperation can begin. Find out as much as possible about the destination you choose and if possible go there in the coolest time of the year. The hospital will probably give you blood-thinning medication such as Warfarin to prevent Deep Vein Thrombosis after the operation and on your long-haul flight, but remember to wear compression socks anyway. You are also advised to take a relative or friend with you, who will usually be allowed to stay in an adjacent bed without charge. It has been proven that familiar faces can help convalescence and prevent loneliness while abroad. Although India now has a huge middle-class population, heart-breaking poverty is everywhere and can come as a shock to some British people.

FARES

Fares to India vary according to the destination city, but as a rule of thumb expect to pay up to £500 for a return ticket in economy class. Look at Middle Eastern carriers like Emirates for some of the best deals.

> While India is rightly famous for its medical tourism, one in every three blind people in the world lives in the country – an estimated 13 million, of which two million are children.
> Every year 2.3 million people develop cataracts, many of which are not treated even though the cost of an operation is as low as $20 (£11.50).

ISRAEL

OFFICIAL NAME: State of Israel
AREA: 20,770 square kilometres (8,019 square miles)
POPULATION: 6,276,883
LANGUAGE: Hebrew
CAPITAL: Jerusalem – but nearly all countries maintain their embassies in Tel Aviv
TIME ZONE: Two hours ahead of Greenwich Mean Time (GMT +2)
DISTANCE: London to Tel Aviv = 3,584 kilometres (2,227 miles)

As one of the world's biggest flashpoints, Israel might not be the first choice for medical tourism, but in fact it has one of the finest medical centres in the world dealing with high-level organ transplants as well as heart and cancer treatments.

RABIN MEDICAL CENTER
(www.clalit.org.il/rabin/Content/Content.asp?CID=73 &u=392)
Jabutinski St, Petah-Tikva, 49100 Israel
Tel: +972 3 9377 377 Fax: +972 3 9376 364
This is the largest medical centre in Israel and it promises to co-ordinate every aspect of the medical tourist's care. The Department of Organ Transplantation performs multi-organ and live donor

liver transplants as well as specialising in kidney and pancreas procedures. It performs transplants for children and the transplant co-ordinator can be contacted on +972 3 9376 473/6.

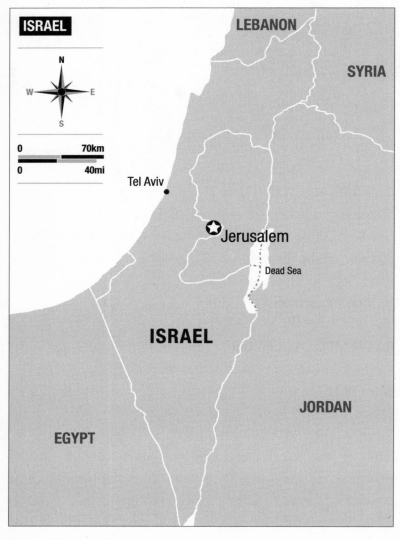

A heart and lung transplant unit is part of the Department of Cardiothoracic Surgery, which performs more than 1,000 heart operations a year. The Institute of Oncology is the largest in Israel and admits about 2,700 new cancer patients a year. It is composed of several units: Outpatient Clinics (18,000 visits per year); Day Care Center for Chemotherapy (about 12,000 annual treatments); the in-hospital ward (20 beds) and the Radiation Therapy Unit (about 200 patients per day). Also available is a psychosocial service, a dietician, stoma nurse and pharmacy unit for the preparation of cytotoxic treatments. The Pulmonary Institute is also one of the largest in Israel, treating complex diseases and critical patients before and after lung transplants.

Medical tourists should enquire directly to the Rabin Medical Center, using the online form, about the cost of high-level treatment.

HEALTH VACATION CENTER LTD
(www.hvc.co.il)
53A Hagefen Street, Ramat Hasharon
Tel: +972 3 5400 135 Fax: +972 3 5401 069
Email: hvc1@netvision.net.il
The HVC pioneered treatment for psoriasis and arthritis at the Dead Sea. Treatment can be over 14, 21 or 28 days and includes regular medical check-ups, ointments and medicines and even the use of physiotherapy and gymnastic facilities.

More than 60,000 patients have been treated at the

clinics and the therapy is based on the climactic factors prevailing at the Dead Sea – the lowest place on the surface of the Earth. The Dead Sea contains about 30 per cent salts with magnesium as the dominating cation and bromide as a dominating anion. Patients who arrived at the Dead Sea with low levels of these ions in the blood were found to have much higher levels after the treatment period. The centre claims 90 per cent of psoriasis patients were clear completely after four weeks of treatment.

For the cost of the different programmes, contact the centre. A convenient registration form is available on the website.

Religious tourism has always been a part of Israel and no visit to the country is really complete without visiting Jerusalem and Bethlehem. But the country's most famous resort has to be Eilat at the southern tip of Israel on the Red Sea. It is heavily built up with hotels to suit every type of budget and is sunny all year round. With its clear waters and coral, it attracts scuba divers and snorkelling fans.

Tel Aviv, the largest city in Israel, is a modern metropolis stretched along an excellent beach strip of the Mediterranean and famous for its seafront skyscrapers. It is also the country's greatest cultural centre, home to a variety of museums, galleries, theatres and concert halls.

FARES

Bucket-shop fares to Tel Aviv are £200–300 return on scheduled airlines. Shop around for charter flights to Eilat.

> The Sheba Medical Center is the largest and most important medical centre in Israel and the Middle East. Situated on a 150–acre campus on the outskirts of Tel Aviv, it has 20 departments and clinics and 1,700 beds. The centre handles 1,117,000 outpatient visits annually and 107,000 inpatients.

ITALY

OFFICIAL NAME: Italian Republic
AREA: 301,230 square kilometres
POPULATION: 58,103,033
LANGUAGE: Italian (official), German and French in small parts of the country
CAPITAL: Rome
TIME ZONE: Central European Time (GMT +1)
DISTANCE: London to Rome = 1,440 kilometres (895 miles)

Italy needs no introduction to anyone who enjoys culture, beautiful women, excellent food and chic cities. But one of the things it's hiding is its reputation as a centre for hair-restoration surgery at very competitive prices, and under the care of doctors who regularly work in the UK.

LASERCOSMEDICS
(http://xoomer.virgilio.it/lasercosmedics/)
Dr Donato Zizi, Laser CosMedics, via Volturno 64020, Scerne di Pineto
Tel: +39 85 946 1049
Email: donatozizi@virgilio.it
The clinic is north of Pescara on Italy's east coast. It offers micro-surgical hair transplants with up to 2,000 grafts in one session and boasts completely natural

results. Prices are £3,000–4,000 (€4,500–6,000). Pity Libya's Colonel Gaddafi didn't know about it. He allegedly got his thatch done in Brazil.

The clinic also offers a range of cosmetic treatments such as:

Lipodissolve therapy for the non-surgical reduction of fat deposits: £200 (€300) per session – usually 4 sessions are required.

Laser removal of thread veins: £300 (€450)

Laser skin resurfacing: £500 (€750)

Botox (1 area): £200 (€300)

Botox (2 areas): £300 (€450)

Botox (3 areas): £380 (€550)

Lip enhancement – lasting up to nine months: £300 (€450)

Glycoclic acid chemical peeling: £100 (€150)

Tricloacetic chemical peeling: £200 (€300)

Cellulite treatment: £100 (€150)

Mole removal: £200 (€300)

From pizza to popes, you get the lot in Italy. Whether you want to visit the heritage sites of Rome or drift down the canals of Venice, there is so much to do and so many places to visit. But if you decide to visit the clinic and stay in the Pescara district, then go in the summer because the city has 10 miles of wide, clean sandy beaches and attracts thousands of Italian families on holiday – although its charms are still a bit of a secret for foreign visitors. It becomes a non-stop

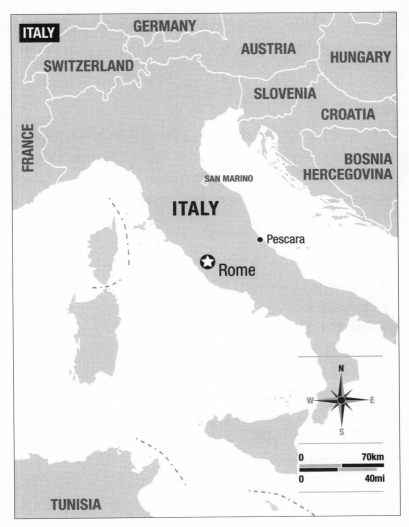

party beach scene when the weather is warm, but in the winter months the city is practically dead. Italians adore eating and Pescara boasts great seafood restaurants and fabulous ice-cream parlours. It's a fairly modern city so there are few historical sights to see, but it has a museum of modern art and the city makes a good jumping-off point for visiting Abruzzo's national parks.

FARES

One of the reasons Pescara is a bit of a secret is because it's fairly expensive to fly there. Both British Airways and British Midland do the route but be prepared to pay between £250 and £400 return. Shop around and book in advance if possible.

HOTELS

It's a holiday town so there are hotels to choose from in all categories.

Top: The Hotel Esplanade at Piazza Primo Maggio, 46 (www.esplanade.net). Tel: +39 85 292141 Fax +39 85 421 7540 Email: reservations@esplanade.net. Rooms £95 (€145) per night. Own stretch of beach.

Middle: The Salus at Lungomare Matteotti, 13. Tel: +39 85 374 196 Fax: +39 85 374 103. Rooms: £44 (€65) per night. On the seafront.

Bottom: The Planet at Via Piave, 142. Tel: +39 85 421 1657. Rooms £34 (€50) per night.

ITALY

Since 1978, Italy has had its own national health service (the SSN or Servizio Sanitario Nazionale). Similar to the British NHS, it is based on the principle of 'universal entitlement', with the State providing free and equal access to preventive medical care and rehabilitation services to all residents.

LATVIA

OFFICIAL NAME: Republic of Latvia
AREA: 64,589 square kilometres (24,938 square miles)
POPULATION: 2,290,237
LANGUAGE: Latvian (official) 58.2 per cent,
Russian 37.5 per cent
CAPITAL: Riga
TIME ZONE: Eastern European Time (GMT +2)
DISTANCE: London to Riga = 1,634 kilometres
(1,016 miles)

Since joining the European Union as a full member in 2004, Latvia – known as 'the pearl of the Baltic States' – has seen a massive increase in tourists from other EU countries and has started catering for them in the area of dental surgery. Free from its communist shackles, the country has flourished and gained a reputation for transforming itself into a market economy, abolishing price controls and initiating privatisation. Medical tourism is now on its agenda.

VILLADENT
(www.villadent.com)
Riga, Dzelzavas 38, LV–1035, Latvia
Fax: +371 757 9809
Email: villa@villadent.com

Villadent specialise in dental services using several dental clinics all over Latvia. They can organise your entire visit and because they have their own dental laboratory they can arrange for crown or bridgework to be done in a weekend. A treatment plan can be arranged and sent to the patient by email so they will know the cost in advance, although payment is not needed until the end of treatment.

The latest equipment is used including intra-oral cameras and digital X-rays, which use 10 times lower radiation than normal X-rays. Here are some approximate procedure costs:

Implant with tooth: €750–1,100 (£500–734)
Teeth whitening: €180 (£120)
Filling with white material: €30 (£20)
Dentures using all ceramic crown: €220 (£147)
Tartar removal using Air Flow system: €35 (£24)

The company can arrange for patients to stay in guest apartments in either of Latvia's two biggest cities – Riga and Daugavpils. Suites in the Riga guesthouse cost €50 (£34) a night with a similar price for a three-room flat in Daugavpils. They also have a catalogue of guesthouses throughout Latvia for patients who want to stay on in the country for a holiday after treatment. They range from €15 (£10) to €100 (£67) a night. A company representative will meet people at the airport and accompany them to where they are staying and to the clinic. If necessary, an interpreter can also be made available during the stay.

The coastal capital of Riga is the most vibrant city of the Baltic countries and is a fairytale mixture of winding streets, church steeples and castles. But it also has some warm and welcoming bars, which are especially homely when the snow is falling. Travel to the west coast and you can visit Liepaja, which has an excellent beach and is rated the hippest town in the country by Latvia's trendsetters thanks to it full-on bars.

If the country doesn't have any world-renowned monuments and attractions, then it makes up for it with the friendliness of its people, especially the young, who are proud of their independent country and love

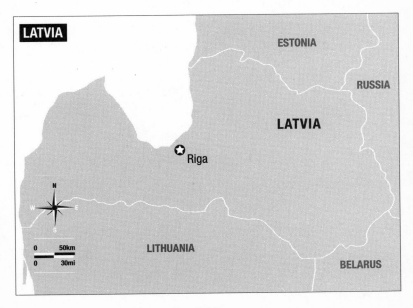

showing it off to tourists. Be prepared to be caught up with a bunch of locals whose hospitality often means you won't be allowed to put your hand in your pocket.

FARES

Expect to pay between £100 and £150 for an economy return to Riga, depending on the carrier and time of year. British Airways, not always the cheapest airline, often do good deals on this route.

> When the iron curtain lifted in the late 1980s and travel outside the Soviet Union became possible, many would-be physicians visited Canada, which is why a great number of Latvian doctors have been trained in Canada and the US and are skilled in the very latest techniques from the West.

MALAYSIA

OFFICIAL NAME: Malaysia

AREA: 329,750 square kilometres (127,317 square miles)

POPULATION: 23,953,136

LANGUAGE: Bahasa Melayu (official), English, Chinese dialects (Cantonese, Mandarin, Hokkien, Hakka, Hainan, Foochow), Tamil, Telugu, Malayalam, Panjabi, Thai

CAPITAL: Kuala Lumpur

TIME ZONE: Greenwich Mean Time plus eight hours (GMT +8)

DISTANCE: London to Kuala Lumpur = 10,552 kilometres (6,557 miles)

Malaysia is fast emerging as a value-for-money destination for health and medical tourism. In 2004, a total of more than 129,000 foreign patients received medical treatment in the country, generating foreign exchange earnings of $27.63 million. Malaysia's health

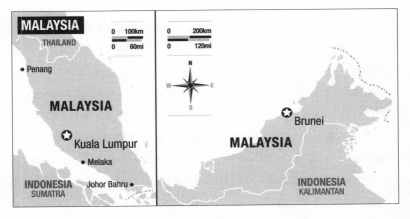

and medical tourism is picking up because of favourable exchange rates and a wide choice of private medical centres with highly qualified medical professionals.

Among the most popularly requested operations are heart-bypass surgery and fertility treatments, plus cosmetic surgery on the island of Penang.

SUNWAY MEDICAL CENTRE
(www.sunway.com.my/sunmed)
No 5, Jalan Lagoon Selatan, Bandar Sunway, 46150 Petaling Jaya, Selangor Darul Ehsan
Tel: +60 3 7491 9191 Fax: + 60 3 7491 8181
Email: smc@sunway.com.my
This is a private hospital offering specialised tertiary healthcare services located in the self-contained township in Selangor Darul Ehsan. The medical complex is an eight-level building with 240 beds and 45 specialist consultation suites. It has all the facilities and services that you would expect of a modern, front-line hospital and is equipped for all medical and surgical disciplines from cancer care to ear, nose and throat surgery.

It is part of an 800-acre 'resort-in-a-city', only 25 minutes from Kuala Lumpur city centre and 35 minutes from the airport. Medical tourists can stay at the five-star Sunway Lagoon Resort Hotel with its 441 rooms, or the popular four-star Pyramid Tower, which has 764 rooms. The medical centre and hotels are adjacent to a gigantic, world-class shopping mall and the Sunway Lagoon theme park.

GORGEOUS GATEWAYS

(http://www.gorgeousgetaways.com/home.htm)
Menara Megah Condo, Block B, Unit 11–23, Jalan
Ipoh Batu 2, Off Jalan Ipoh 51200, Kuala Lumpur
Tel: +60 3 4045 1498
Email: info@gorgeousgateways.com

Gorgeous Gateways are independent operators that
tailor medical tourism packages to Malaysia. They offer
both cosmetic and holistic treatments, and boast, 'We
provide all the arrangements and services so you don't
have to do anything. From all pre-surgery advice and
consultation, to transfers and representation at the
hospital and hotel, we will be there for you so you don't
have to worry about a thing.'

Here are examples of some of their all-inclusive
packages (return flights from UK not included). All
prices are approximate, and depend on individual needs.
Breast enlargement: £2,400. Includes: private hospital
fees, anaesthetist, theatre and surgery, pathology, X-
ray fees; one night in a single, private room at the
hospital; all-inclusive treatments, eg implants,
bandages, dressings; any prescribed medications; 24-
hour on-call post-operative care; pre- and post-
surgery consultations by leading surgeon, as
necessary; 10 nights' package accommodation in a
five-star luxury hotel; all transfers to and from the
hospital, airport and hotel. If you prefer a luxury
apartment to a hotel, the price drops to £1,960 and a
second person can stay free.

Full facelift: £1,600. Includes same five-star hotel package as breast enlargement.

Liposuction to hips, thighs and buttocks: £1,500 for the five-star package.

Laser teeth whitening: £270

Porcelain veneers or crowns: £150 each

LASIK sight correction (both eyes): £760

Because of the holistic approach offered, the company can also arrange fitness, diet and nutrition, and massage and pampering treatments. A personal fitness trainer can be included in your package and you can select how many sessions you would like.

BEAUTIFUL HOLIDAYS
(www.beautiful holidays.com/ver2/services/intro/intro.asp)
34 Nagore Road, 10050 Georgetown, Penang
Tel: +60 4 227 9010 Fax: +60 4 227 5857
Email: admin@beautiful-holidays.com
They are similar to Gorgeous Gateways, but are based in Penang and have a selection of four hotels and two clinics. They specialise in all the major cosmetic surgeries including ear reshaping, tummy tucks and breast reduction as well as eye surgery, and prices are available on application.

HOTELS
The Paradise Sandy Bay: Located on the beach in

Tanjung Bunga about 10 minutes' drive from the city. Good four-star hotel with large rooms.

The Lone Pine Hotel: Beach-based in the holiday area of Batu Ferringhi, but in a quiet location for peaceful recovery.

Eastern and Oriental Hotel: Five-star colonial splendour on the waterfront, within walking distance of the city centre.

Golden Sands Hotel: Five-star hotel in Batu Ferringhi.

Discerning tourists combine a week at the Eastern and Oriental for luxurious recovery with a second week on the beach in the Golden Sands.

MAHKOTA MEDICAL CENTRE, MELAKA

(http://www.hmi.com.sg/hc/mmc.htm)
No 3, Mahkota Melaka, Jalan Merdeka, 75000 Melaka
Tel: +60 6 281 3333 Fax: +60 6 281 0560
Email: info@mahkotamedical.com

A 238-bed hospital offering homely hostel rooms in the same block for visiting family members. The centre's specialities include open-heart surgery. Outpatients might want to consider Mahkota's three-day/two-night health-screening packages, which include tours of the historic town and even transportation to a local golf course.

COUNTRY HEIGHTS MEDICAL TOURISM, KUALA LUMPUR

The country's only medical screening centre within a five-star resort, Country Heights Medical Tourism offer patients a battery of diagnostic tests (including fluoroscopy and abdominal ultrasounds), and the results five hours later. Pass the time by taking a water taxi to the neighbouring Mines Shopping Fair for a bout of retail therapy.

DAMANSARA FERTILITY CENTRE
http://www.damansarafertility.com/
There are three centres:
No 55 Jalan SS 21/56B, Damansara Utama, 47400
Petaling Jaya, Selangor, Malaysia
Tel: +60 3 7729 3199 Fax: +60 3 7727 8066
No 8 Jalan Prima, Metro Prima, Kepong,
52100 Kuala Lumpur
Tel: +60 3 6258 0000
Unit 18, Level 1, City Plaza, No 21 Jalan Tebrau,
60300 Johor Bahru
Tel: +60 7 278 0088 Fax: +60 7 278 0808.

The clinics offer all the usual fertility services and procedures plus a lot more, like sex selection, assisted hatching and even surrogacy. The centre is nearly 12 years old, and in 2004 announced Malaysia's first Freeze Thaw Blastocyst delivery with a baby boy weighing in at 3.45kg. It deals with couples from all parts of the world including the UK – a British woman had twins, born 18 months apart – with a high success rate. Contact the centres for costs and availability.

Malaysia is a wonder, and not just because it has the world's tallest building with the twin Petronas Towers in Kuala Lumpur – although don't miss the observation deck – but because, for an Asian country, it is fairly hassle-free. When the relentless cosmopolitan bustle of modern KL starts to get to you, there is an escape in the botanical and bird parks of the Lake Gardens. Malacca, 150 kilometres (93 miles) south of KL, is the antithesis of the capital city. The seaside city is much quieter and steeped in history. Penang offers outstanding beaches as well as the largest temple complex in Southeast Asia at Air Itam.

Malyasia is hot and humid all year round, and you need to get acclimatised to the weather, with the rainy season on the peninsula's east coast from November to January.

FARES
Return flights to Kuala Lumpur using schedule airlines like KLM or Air Lanka should cost around £500 return in economy. But expect to pay £600 plus if you're going to Penang.

As well as offering medical procedures, Malaysia's promotion of health tourism, which started in 1997, also includes activities that enhance health such as trekking, cycling, jogging and swimming, along with health screening and massages at spas set up all around the country.

MEXICO

OFFICIAL NAME: United Mexican States
AREA: 1,972,550 square kilometres (761,606 square miles)
POPULATION: 106,202,903
LANGUAGE: Spanish, various Mayan, Nahuatl and other regional indigenous languages
CAPITAL: Mexico (Distrito Federal)
TIME ZONE: Greenwich Mean Time minus six hours (GMT −6)
DISTANCE: London to Mexico City = 8,898 kilometres (5,529 miles)

For years Americans have been travelling over the border into Mexico for every kind of medical treatment from alternative cancer cures in Tijuana to body sculpting in the resort areas. With the rise in package-deal holidays to Mexico, British travellers are discovering there is more to this Central American country than the hedonistic beaches of Acapulco.

The tourist hotspot of Cabo San Lucas, on the tip of Baja California Sur, is fast becoming a centre for medical tourism. While Cabo nightlife is not on a par with Acapulco, the town attracts a young, energetic crowd to clubs like Squid Roe and Giggling Marlin that creates a more vibrant ambiance than is found at the relatively laid-back city of San José to the north.

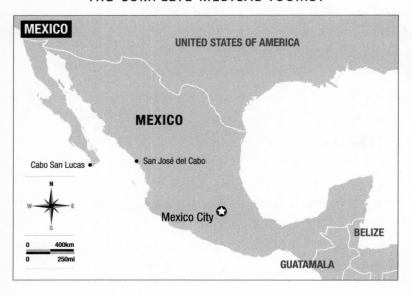

MIGUELANGELO PLASTIC SURGERY CLINIC

(http://miguelangeloclinic.com)

Hotel Hacienda Beach Resort, Int #6,

Cabo San Lucas, Baja California Sur, Mexico

Tel: +52 624 143 4303 Fax: +52 624 143 4391

Email: info@miguelangeloclinic.com

The clinic provides excellent patient recovery because it is located on the premises of a fashionable beach resort. It has a state-of-the-art surgery suite with private recovery room and 24-hour nurse care. The staff carries out all treatments and procedures indicated under Cosmetic Surgery in Section One of this handbook, and the first night of post-operative recovery at the Hotel Hacienda, with rooms overlooking the Sea of Cortez, is included in the medical cost.

ANGELS TOUCH DENTAL CLINIC

(http://www.angelsdental.com)
Plazas Doradas Building local #7,
San José del Cabo, Mexico
Tel: +52 624 142 6192
Email: info@angelsdental.com

Arranges for discounted hotel rooms for patients wanting dental treatment. Dr Rosa Pena, the smile designer (well, this is the Americas), claims you can pay for your Mexican holiday because prices are so cheap. Two root canals and two crowns cost $1,600 (£900).

'Angels Touch Clinics can save you serious money on your cosmetic dentistry. It is not unusual for entire families to schedule a trip to Los Cabos with parents and children all visiting our dental clinic together. Seniors, who have more time than money (and more need of a dentist), often enjoy the greatest savings on their larger treatments,' she says.

There are three clinics. Cabo San Lucas and San José del Cabo are holiday spots with five-star hotels, golf courses, fine restaurants, art galleries and serious big-game fishing. More than two million tourists visit the area annually. Los Barriles is 40 minutes north and, years ago, was the secret hideaway where many Hollywood stars like John Wayne, Bing Crosby, Desi Arnez and others would arrive by private yacht or small plane to do serious big-game fishing.

The Baja peninsula is one of the most interesting and diverse geographical areas of the world and is still very much a frontier. The peninsula is home to some of Earth's most beautiful deserts, along with semi-tropical and mountainous regions, pine forests, and hundreds of miles of untouched beaches and coastline. Most people of mainland Mexico consider it a far-off place, much in the way Americans would think of Alaska – distant, mystical, harsh and beautiful. Although a frontier, it is a popular destination for travellers, especially those from all over North America seeking warm weather in the winter months. Its tropical desert environment next to the sea makes the Baja peninsula warm all year round. The hottest period is July to November, which is when the hotel rates are lowest. There is a hurricane season, which runs from mid-September to mid-October – hurricanes don't strike every year, but when they do it can be an adventure.

FARES

The main airport on Baja California Sur is Gen de Leon at La Paz, north of the peninsula tip. Prices can be high because you will have to change planes. Try American Airlines and expect to pay £600+ for economy return. The German carrier Lufthansa can be £100 cheaper, so shop around. An internal flight can be taken from La Paz down to San José del Cabo.

Many North Americans now travel to Mexico for dental work and minor surgery, as prices are considerably lower. Pharmaceuticals are widely available and at prices much lower than in the US or Canada. Doctors are well trained and they even do house calls! Mexican people are generally friendly and helpful. They almost always return a greeting, and usually with a smile.

POLAND

OFFICIAL NAME: Republic of Poland
AREA: 312,685 square kilometres (120,728 square miles)
POPULATION: 38,635,144
LANGUAGE: Polish
CAPITAL: Warsaw
TIME ZONE: Central European Time (GMT +1)
DISTANCE: London to Warsaw = 1,467 kilometres
(912 miles)

Poland could not have wished for better publicity about its emerging medical-tourist industry than when, last year, Blanche from *Coronation Street* decided to go to Gdansk to have her hip operation rather than wait for months on the National Health Service. Forget her somewhat grumpy recovery – that's called dramatic licence. What she did do was introduce the idea of medical tourism to millions of viewers. And prices in Poland are astonishingly good value. German medical tourists were the first to realise the value that could be had in Poland and the number of German patients is doubling every year. But now that Poland is part of the European Union the pace of medical tourism has started to increase with more and more people from Britain choosing to have treatment in the country.

DAMIAN MEDICAL CENTER

(http://www.damian.com.pl/english/)

46 Walbrzyska Str (near Sluzew station), Warsaw

Tel: +48 22 566 2222

Email: turystyka@damian.com.pl

This was the first private hospital in the Polish capital. It was established in 1994 and the medical team are fluent in English. There are 40 hospital beds and three operating theatres designed and equipped to European Union standards.

Here are examples of some of the centre's prices for

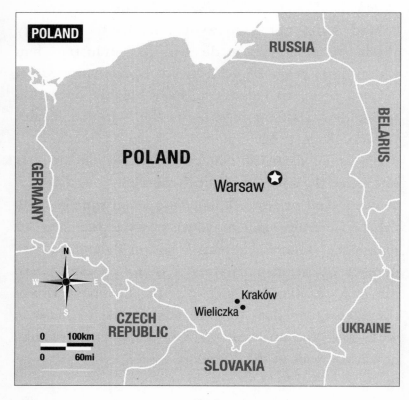

the more popular procedures, which include the cost of hospitalisation but not convalescence.

COSMETIC
Face and neck wrinkles: €1,227–2,182 (£818–1,455)
Ear correction: €545–818 (£363–545)
Nose correction: €955–1,773 (£637–1,182)
Breast reduction: €1,364–2,455 (£909–1,637)
**Breast enlargement (without
   prostheses):** €1,227–1,636 (£818–1,091)
Liposuction: €818–1,909 (£545–1,273)
Hair transplant: €955–1,636 (£637–1,091)
Botox: €280–850 (£187–567)
DENTAL
One implant: €1,400 (£934)
Porcelain crown: €200–400 (£133–266)
GENERAL SURGERY
Hernia: €641 (£427)
Haemorrhoids: €736 (£491)
Varicose veins: €518–1,173 (£345–782)

Convalescence is offered at the four-star Villa Park Hotel in the Ciechocinek health resort in central Poland. There are apartments as well as rooms for the disabled plus restaurant and bar. The facility, being a health and beauty clinic, also offers a choice of treatments, including a swimming pool, brine Jacuzzi baths with access to a 'wet bar', hydrotherapy, balneotherapy, treatments in the Alphamassage capsule, steam baths, sessions in an oxygen bar, sessions in a cryochamber, and treatments at the beauty salon and Face and Body Aesthetics Salon. For more information about the hotel, plus prices, log on to www.villapark.pl.

BARBARA THURGOOD & COMPANY, MEDICAL SERVICES
(www.barbarathurgood.com/welcome_page.htm)
9 Ridge Langley, South Croydon, Surrey CR2 0AP, UK
Tel: 020 8651 5443
Email: info@barbarathurgood.com
This company has been organising fixed-price surgery packages to Krakow in Poland since 1995. For knee, hip and shoulder replacement, they offer 28-day complete packages, which include diagnosis, treatment at the Jagiellonian University Orthopaedic Hospital and Rehabilitation Centre in Krakow, plus physiotherapy. It is a fully escorted service, with the patient collected and taken to Gatwick Airport and a night's stay at a Gatwick hotel if so desired. The patient will be escorted all the way to Krakow so that it's not necessary to involve family or friends unless so wished. English-speaking co-ordinators are on hand all the time at the hospital for personal shopping, laundry and sightseeing excursions around Krakow at the end of the stay. The hospital is situated in a quiet, residential part of Krakow. The single and double rooms are all en-suite with Sky TV, private telephone line and nurses on call 24 hours a day. Special dietary requirements are also catered for.

POLAND

Here are some of the orthopaedic package prices:
Total knee replacement: £5,950 (28-day stay)
Total hip replacement: £5,950 (28-day stay)
Knee arthroscopy: £3,750 (14-day stay)
Knee revision: £7,950 (28-day stay)
Hip revision: £7,950 (28-day stay)
Shoulder replacement: £5,950 (28-day stay)

The company can also arrange comprehensive cosmetic-surgery packages, which include the surgical procedure, all nursing care, return flights from the UK and all transfers, plus post-operative consultation in the UK. For the six-day package, you get five nights' full-board accommodation and, for the 11-day package, 10 nights' full-board.

Here is an example of some package deal prices:
Breast augmentation: £2,500 (6 days); £2,900
  (11 days)
Breast reduction: £3,100 (6 days); £3,500 (11 days)
Gynaecomastia: £2,000; £2,400
Breast uplift: £3,000; £3,400
Ear correction: £1,900; £2,300
Upper and lower eyelids: £1,900; £2,300
Facelift (including neck lift): £3,200; £3,600
Rhinoplasty: £2.600; £3,000
Liposuction: from £2,150
Botox: from £250

Dental treatment can also be arranged with the same sort of package but with shorter stays. Here are examples:

Veneer: £390 (2–4 days)
Teeth whitening: £490 (1 day)
All ceramic crown: £450 (2–4 days)
Two dental implants fitted with two ball attachments and removable denture: £3,400 (first visit – 3 days; second visit – 5 days)
Three dental implants fitted with a cylinder bar between them and permanent denture: £5,545 (first visit – 3 days; second visit – 5 days)

Barbara Thurgood & Co also arrange cataract and varicose-vein treatment as well as low-dose CT scans.

WIELICZKA SALT MINE
(www.wieliczka.pl/english/index.html)
Ul Danilowicza 10 32-020, Wieliczka, Poland
Tel: +48 12 278 7302
Email: urystyka@kopalnia.pl
Situated 10 kilometres (6 miles) to the east of Krakow, the salt mine is accessible from Krakow's main railway station. Respiratory diseases, asthma, allergies and skin diseases can all be treated during a six-and-a-half-hour visit to the Lake Wessel Chamber located 135 metres (443 feet) underground, which boasts physical therapy equipment. The special

microclimate in the chamber is bacteriologically pure, with large quantities of sodium chloride and magnesium and calcium ions.

Comprehensive deals including accommodation and full board in hotels near to the mine can be arranged. As an example, you could have a 17-night stay in a hotel with 14 daily visits to the mine's chamber, plus a guided trip of the town and transfers to and from the airport during the 2006 summer season (starting on 27 March) for around £845 per person (double room full board), or for £1,000 for a single.

Poland is rapidly shaking off the restraints of communism and nowhere is it more apparent than in the capital, Warsaw, where old buildings have given way to modern skyscrapers. The city is divided into two parts by the Wisla River, with most of the tourist attractions on the left side. The Old Town is the most attractive part of Warsaw with its quaint, cobbled streets and unique architecture dating back to the 13th century. There are excellent restaurants, cafés and shops in the area. The New Town is located between Krasinskiego Street in the north, Dluga Street to the south, Adama Mickiewicza Street in the west and Wybrzeze Gdanskie Street in the east. It is a pedestrian's haven and mostly closed to traffic. The Jewish Ghetto, which had a population of more than 400,000 before they were almost entirely sent to the Nazi death camps, is filled with monuments and memorials to the people and worth visiting.

Krakow came through the Second World War unscathed and is a major tourist destination, often referred to as 'the new Prague'. The Old Town is a World Heritage Site and one of the best medieval city centres in Europe. Its cathedral is the spiritual home of Poland. Just walking around Krakow is a magical experience with its mix of pavement cafés and market stalls.

FARES

Bucket-shop economy return fares to either Warsaw or Krakow can be as low as £100. Search around and don't expect to pay more than £150 maximum.

> The emergency number in Poland is the same as the UK – 999. But don't rely on anyone answering in English and sadly the public health sector is nowhere nears as good as the private sector. So, if you do have a minor ailment or injury during your post-op holiday, you'll have to pay again.

SOUTH AFRICA

OFFICIAL NAME: Republic of South Africa

AREA: 1,219,912 square kilometres (758,018 square miles)

POPULATION: 44,344,136

LANGUAGE: IsiZulu 23.8 per cent, IsiXhosa 17.6 per cent, Afrikaans 13.3 per cent, Sepedi 9.4 per cent, English 8.2 per cent, Setswana 8.2 per cent, Sesotho 7.9 per cent, Xitsonga 4.4 per cent

CAPITAL: Pretoria

TIME ZONE: Greenwich Mean Time plus two hours (GMT +2)

DISTANCE: London to Johannesburg = 9,067 kilometres (5,634 miles)

London to Cape Town = 9,674 kilometres (6,011 miles)

South Africa is one of the fastest-growing tourist destinations in the world, and medical tourism has not been left out. Thanks to world-class surgeons and an exchange rate that is still favourable, you can winter in the warmth of the Cape and literally come back a different person – because both cosmetic surgery and dentistry are major draws in South Africa.

Hospitals in the Western Cape, such as Tygerberg and Groote Shuur, claim they would love to be allowed to treat NHS patients from the UK, but European Union laws have to be changed before this can happen. So, more and more private patients are flying there themselves. South Africa is a vast country packed with attractions, but the majority of medical tourists seem to prefer going to Johannesburg and Cape Town for their surgery, before maybe going on safari.

Surgeon & Safari
(www.surgeon-and-safari.co.za/)
PO Box 97646, Petervale, 2151, South Africa
Tel: +27 11 463 3154 Fax +27 11 706 5582
Email: info@surgeon-and-safari.co.za
This is probably the most famous medical tourism facility in South Africa for cosmetic surgery, and was established by Lorraine Melvill.

The service offers to co-ordinate all medical correspondence with your selected surgeon; prepare

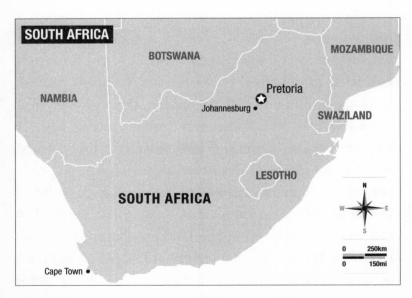

detailed cost estimates; arrange all medical consultations; assist in your preparation for surgery, accommodation and safari; make all necessary bookings, and accompany you to your surgery and medical appointments.

Half of Melvill's clients come from the UK and half from the USA; they stay at The Westcliff Hotel in Johannesburg or The Cellars-Hohenort Hotel in Cape Town for one or two weeks' recovery before going on safari.

Although the company is famous for arranging every type of cosmetic surgery from facelifts to laser skin resurfacing and hair transplants, it can also provide all forms of eye surgery, orthopaedic procedures and dentistry as well as sports-injury treatments.

For recuperation, The Westcliff Hotel in Johannesburg is perched on a hillside overlooking the city's zoological gardens and is favoured by celebrities and statesmen from all over the world. The Cellars-Hohenort in Cape Town is situated in the secure Constantia Valley. A private guesthouse with a swimming pool is also available for people who hanker after more privacy.

And safaris are not just confined to trekking out into the bush. There are wine safaris, where you can taste some of South Africa's finest tipples, and a train safari from Cape Town to Pretoria and back on the world's most luxurious locomotive, The Blue Train, which has all the comfort of a five-star hotel. Obviously, going on safari after recuperation does not make for the cheapest form of medical tourism in the world, but it may still prove better value than having a single procedure performed in the UK.

Here are some of their prices for treatment only, many of which require between seven and twelve days' recuperation:

COSMETIC
Ear repair: £1,300
Brow lift: £1,730
Breast augmentation: £2,300
Breast lift: £2,650
Breast reduction: £2,650
Eyelid surgery: £1,800
Facelift: £3,600
Nose surgery: £2,200
Tummy tuck: £2,650
Botox: £150

DENTAL
Crowns per tooth: £427
Veneers per tooth: £409
Implants per tooth: £654
Bleaching: £409
Full upper and lower denture set: £500

OPHTHALMIC
LASIK (both eyes): £1,400
Cataract (per eye): £1,600

The costs of accommodation, which include transfers to and from the airport and to medical appointments, are as follows:

The Westcliff Hotel, Johannesburg (10 days): £2,272

The Cellars-Hohenort Hotel, Cape Town (10 days): £2,545

Guesthouse (10 days): £1,681 (per room)

Guesthouse (10 days): £1,190 (en-suite per person)

A young lady from the UK who had cosmetic surgery performed by Dr Dirk Lazarus in Cape Town, South Africa, wrote back to the surgeon, 'Just a quick update on how things have been since my return to the UK. After the initial worries about the prolonged swelling to my face and slightly distorted lips I am happy to report that they have now settled down (as you reassuringly said they would) and the result and accompanying comments from friends and family have been wonderful. They were all complimentary about the naturalness of the look, so I have been dishing out your name to all who have been praising your work. In fact "Doing a Dirk" has become an affectionate synonym for any questions they have about their own potential for future surgical procedures, or merely to clandestinely ask if someone they know has "Done a Dirk". On the lipo-body/thigh front there is a marked improvement in my silhouette and the fit of my clothes, so I will definitely be returning some time next year to see if you can sculpt things a little more and to see if you can work a little more of your "magic", especially to the "flank" hip area.'

NU LOOK SURGERY

(www.nulooksurgery.com/index.shtml)
Tel: +27 21 791 4111
Email: Info@nulooksurgery.com

They offer cosmetic and eye surgery in Cape Town with an initial consultation in the UK before travelling to South Africa. They can organise very flexible accommodation from self-catering to five-star luxury, as well as provide a chauffeur, nursing care during recovery and other travel advice. They advise patients to be in Cape Town two or three days before surgery so that consultations can be arranged.

Here is an example of some of their prices. They include pre-consultation, treatment, two nights in a clinic or hospital, private nurse, airport transfers, private chauffeur and post-consultation. They do not include return fares to Cape Town or the cost of hotel accommodation:

Breast enlargement:	£2,269	10-day stay
Mini facelift:	£2,489	10-day stay
Full facelift (including neck):	£3,472	10-day stay
Upper and lower eyelids:	£1,832	7-day stay
Breast reduction:	£2,472	10-day stay
Tummy tuck:	£3,032	14-day stay
LASIK (both eyes):	£1,182	7-day stay
Rhinoplasty:	£2,120	10-day stay

Accommodation can be arranged, although the patient is under no obligation to take it. Typically, a 10-day stay in a four-star guesthouse with breakfast will cost about £287. They offer five-, four- and three-star hotels, health spas, self-catering apartments and houses, and bed and breakfast. The company is also a licensed credit broker offering secure and unsecured loans. One of the four-star guesthouses they recommend is Celtic Manor, which is situated on Steenbras Mountain with views across False Bay to Table Mountain, and overlooks Bikini Beach and Gordon's Bay Yacht Club.

MEDISCAPES SURGERY ABROAD
(www.surgeryabroad.com)
42 Burg Street, Cape Town, South Africa 8000
Tel: +27 21 422 3932 Fax: +27 21 422 3937
Email: info@mediscapes.com
They deal with every possible medical procedure and treatment you can think of – and then some – from alcohol and drug addictions to kidney transplants and brain surgery, as well as the usual cosmetic and dentistry. Their website is one of the best around.

They also offer a Forever Fabulous package at the five-star luxury Twelve Apostles Hotel on the edge of the Atlantic Ocean in Cape Town. The hotel has everything you would expect from one that has been consistently voted in the top 100 in the world – including a butler on call 24 hours a day and a personal shopper. It boasts seven treatment rooms for hydrotherapy, tanning and massage as well as an outdoor swimming pool flanked by two Jacuzzis.

Here are some prices, which can fluctuate depending on the exchange rate. Return flights from the UK and accommodation are not included:

Facelift:	$6,613 (£3,673)	10-night stay
Rhinoplasty:	$5,022 (£2,790)	10-night stay
Breast augmentation:	$5,990 (£3,327)	10-night stay
LASIK surgery:	$3,818 (£2,121)	7-night stay
Hair transplants:	$6,992 (£3,884)	5- to 10-day stay
Infertility IVF/ICSI:	$11,506 (£6,392)	14-night stay
Dental laser whitening:	$558 (£310)	same day
Botox:	$365 (£203)	same day

Mediscapes uses a variety of private hospitals and clinics including the medi-clinic group; this has hospitals like the Panorama on the lower slopes of the Tygerberg Hills in Cape Town, is equipped with CT and MRI scanners, and offers a specialist cardiology centre.

The Louis Leipoldt medi-clinic is located in the city of Bellville in the north of the greater Cape Town area. Here, clients can undergo procedures and surgery that range from dermatology, plastic and reconstructive surgery, ear, nose and throat surgery, maxillofacial and oral surgery, and orthopaedic procedures.

Apart from the elite Twelve Apostles Hotel, the company can offer standard three-star and luxury four-star packages. You should contact them for the latest offers and prices.

Following recovery there is also the option of a safari or visit to a game lodge; a visit to the teeming metropolis of Johannesburg, or even a holiday on one of the Indian Ocean's famous island resorts like Mauritius or Zanzibar.

SURGICAL ATTRACTIONS
(www.surgicalattractions.com)
45 Bristol Road, Parkwood, Johannesburg 2193, South Africa
Tel: +27 11 880 5122 Fax: +27 11 788 9043
Email: info@surgicalattractions.com
Surgical Attractions use a number of top hospitals in both Johannesburg and Cape Town. They specialise in dental, ophthalmic and cosmetic procedures, and recommend surgeons to you after you have forwarded your medical history and set out what you desire for the outcome of the treatment. They claim this personalises treatment and prevents clients from becoming victims of one-size-fits-all surgery. Various medical facilities are used, including the top-rated Kingsbury Hospital in Cape Town and the Donald Gordon Medical Centre in Johannesburg.

Recuperation can take place in a variety of luxury hotels, including the Saxon in Johannesburg where Nelson Mandela chose to relax and edit his autobiography *Long Walk To Freedom*.

The Highlands Hotel in Cape Town once played host to Sherlock Holmes author Arthur Conan Doyle and has been fully restored for visitors to enjoy the hospitality of a bygone age.

Post-recovery holidays include safaris, dynamic train journeys, and country and coastal tours.

Testimonials from satisfied UK clients are available on the stylish website and prices for individual treatments can be acquired by contacting the company by email.

Here is an example of some surgery prices:

Breast augmentation: £2,060–£2,145
Chin implants: £1,370–1,460
Facelift: £3,175–3,860
Botox: £190
Otoplasty: £1,030–1,115
Hair transplant: £1,200–3,090 (the individual client has to be assessed for his true requirements)
Abdominoplasty: £1,630–1,930
Rhinoplasty: £1,715–2,016
Eyelid lift: £945–1,630
Laser eye surgery: £1,160
Lip augmentation: £290–585
Liposuction (for all areas of the body): £1,975–2,060

Even if you don't decide to go on safari or take any of the other tours offered by some of the operators, there is still plenty to see in Cape Town. With the breathtaking backdrop of Table Mountain and its wonderful beaches, it is one of the most picture-postcard perfect places in the world' because it is where old and new converge.

The most glamorous beach is probably Clifton which has four adjoining coves and plenty of luxurious bungalows, but don't miss out on the trendy Camps Bay or the small and romantic Llandudno Beach. There is a lively music scene of all types in the city and the whole place has a relaxed atmosphere. And although crime is on the way down the usual precautions apply about keeping your wits about you and not going out with too much cash.

Johannesburg, about 1,600 kilometres to the north, is the financial and economic capital and is a bit overwhelming because it is so big and flat. There are plenty of no-go areas and it is best to stick to the affluent northern suburbs with their American-style shopping malls.

FARES

Cape Town is serviced by most of the major airlines and return economy bucket-shop prices can be as low as £400 depending on the time of year you want to fly. But expect to pay around £500 on average, and be aware that this can rise considerably in UK wintertime. Prices are very similar for Johannesburg.

High-quality tap water is available almost everywhere in South Africa. It's treated to be free of harmful micro-organisms and is palatable and safe to drink straight from the tap, although beware of trying it in shack settlements. Bottled water is also readily available.

SPAIN

OFFICIAL NAME: Kingdom of Spain
AREA: 499,542 square kilometres (192,874 square miles)
POPULATION: 40,341,462
LANGUAGE: Castilian Spanish
CAPITAL: Madrid
TIME ZONE: Central European Time (GMT +1)
DISTANCE: London to Barcelona = 1,146 kilometres
(712 miles)

Best known for its sun and sangria, Spain is slowly getting a reputation for its cosmetic surgery as well. It is a favourite holiday destination and retirement spot for British citizens and one of the European Union's great success stories, having economically rocketed since the downfall of dictator General Franco. The Spanish people are so happy with the EU that when they were allowed to vote on its proposed constitution in February 2005 they overwhelmingly supported it, even though France and subsequently Holland rejected the idea, shunting the constitution into the sidings.

More than 50 million people a year visit Spain from all over the world to enjoy its long sandy beaches, its superb old buildings from Gothic cathedrals to awe-inspiring palaces, and its fantastic galleries packed with works by its great painters such as Picasso, El Greco,

Dali and Goya. Now those tourists can come back with more than just a smile on their face.

Cosmetic Surgery Abroad
(www.cosmeticsurgeryabroad.org)
c/ Escuelas Pias 103, 08017 Barcelona
Tel/Fax: +34 932 54 5411
Email: drbenito@cirugia-estetica.com
They also have consultations in the UK. They can be contacted through Cosmedicate at 122 Harley Street, London W1G 7JP (Tel: 020 7224 1010) and at St John's Street, Manchester M3 4FA (Tel: 016 1907 2601). Customers should phone or email to find out when the surgeon will be visiting the UK cities. The first consultation in the UK is free of charge.

They offer all the usual cosmetic surgical procedures

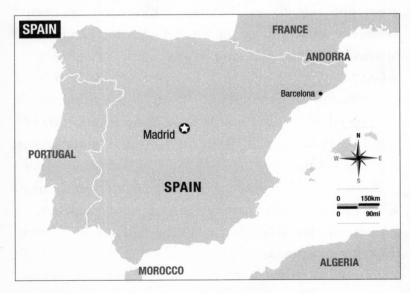

as well as enhancing calves, chins and body contouring for men. They advise a stay in Barcelona of at least four to ten days after surgery, depending on the treatment, and suggest that any sightseeing in the city is done before the operation, as after surgery patients will need to rest in a relaxed environment to recover quickly. Dissolving stitches are used in most procedures, so there is no need to stay in Barcelona to remove them and a follow-up visit is done in London.

Prices include all treatment and hospital stay, plus transfers from the airport. Flights to Barcelona are not included:

Tummy tuck with liposuction:	£3,800	(4-day stay)
Breast augmentation:	£3,500	(2-day stay)
Gynaecomastia:	£2,400	(2-day stay)
Eyelids (two lids):	£1,400	(1-day stay)
Neck and facelift:	£3,800	(3-day stay)
Buttock augmentation:	£3,500	(3-day stay)
Facelift plus eyes:	£4,800	(4-day stay)
Liposuction abdomen:	£2,400	(2-day stay)
Ear surgery:	£1,400	(1-day stay)
Pectoral implants for men:	£5,000	(2-day stay)
Liposuction arms:	£2,100	(1-day stay)
Breast lift:	£3,500	(3-day stay)
Breast lift or augmentation with tummy tuck:	£6,000	(4-day stay)
Breast reduction:	£3,800	(3-day stay)
Nose surgery:	£2,400	(2-day stay)

HOTELS

Here are some of the hotels the company recommends for people who want to stay longer in the city:

Three-star: Hotel Mikado, Tel: +34 932 114 166 Fax: 932114210, in the medical, business and residential area of the city, has 68 en-suite rooms all with air-conditioning, satellite TV and minibar. The hotel has a restaurant, coffee bar and other facilities.

Four-star: Hotel Hesperia Sarriá (). Tel: +34 932 045 551 Fax: +34 932 044 392. Situated in the residential area of Tres Torres, the hotel has 138 fully equipped rooms, is 4 kilometres (2.5 miles) from the city centre and 7 kilometres (4 miles) from the beach.

For costs of procedures and hotels, contact Cosmetic Surgery Abroad.

Barcelona is probably the trendiest and most fashionable city on the Mediterranean. The city's most famous area is Las Ramblas, a tree-lined pedestrian boulevard of five separate streets strung end-to-end and selling everything from birds to lottery tickets. It also has strip clubs and peep clubs, and can be loud and eye-poppingly entertaining. Sadly, Barcelona is also the pickpocket capital of the Med, so hang on to your belongings and never go out with too much cash or too many credit cards in your wallet.

The city's beaches are clean but crowded in the season, especially Nova Icaria, the closest one to the

Olympic marina. It is impossible to miss the surrealistically warped Gothic architecture of Antonio Gaudi. The champion of Spanish Art Nouveau is liked and loathed in equal doses, but he can't be dismissed. If you see only one Gaudi building, make it the Sagrada Familia. This cathedral is really only a facade because Gaudi died before he could see it completed, but it is a landmark of modern architecture and is still being constructed to this day.

FARES
Shop around and you should be able to get an economy return flight to Barcelona for around £100. But expect to pay more in the peak summer season.

Although it is perfectly safe, many people find the tap water in Barcelona a bit distasteful because of its high mineral content, so it's advisable to go for bottled. And the high humidity and noticeable levels of air pollution tend to make the flu and other respiratory diseases common in the city.

THAILAND

OFFICIAL NAME: Kingdom of Thailand
AREA: 514,000 square kilometres 198,456.5
POPULATION: 65,444,371
LANGUAGE: Thai, English (secondary language of the elite)
CAPITAL: Bangkok
TIME ZONE: Greenwich Mean Time plus seven hours (GMT +7)
DISTANCE: London to Bangkok = 9,540 kilometres (5,928 miles)

Thailand was probably the first of the major medical tourist destinations, thanks in many ways to its currency collapsing in 1997. The hospitals decided they needed to lure Western patients and they did so with low prices, modern facilities and beautiful beaches. Since then, things have mushroomed and Thailand is a leading country for cosmetic surgery as well as the world's number-one place for gender reassignment, also known as a 'sex change'. There are literally scores – if not hundreds – of sex-change clinics in Thailand. The modern hospitals for medical tourism are usually situated in resort areas, and offer top-class dining and even tourist souvenirs.

It was feared the tsunami that struck parts of Thailand on Boxing Day 2004 might have destroyed the medical-tourist market, but business has proved more resilient.

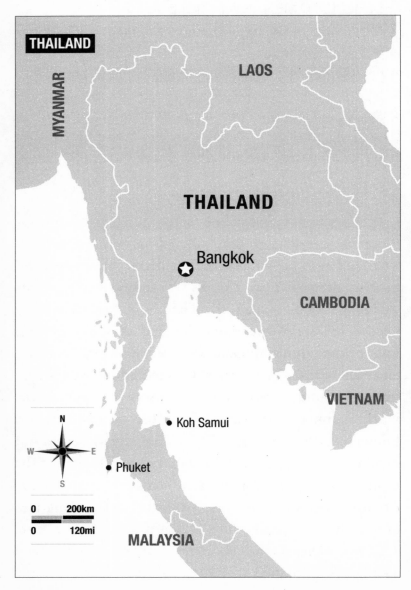

PHUKET HEALTH AND TRAVEL

(http://www.phuket-health-travel.com/)

2/1 Hongsyok Utis Road, Samkong, Phuket 83000, Thailand

Tel: +66 76 354 055 Fax: +66 76 354 056

Email: info@phuket-health-travel.com

They offer just about everything from delivering your baby to changing your sex, as well as organising package deals for certain procedures. Their extraordinarily detailed website even has a Skype contact, Ulf Mikaelsson, for people using Voice Over Internet Protocol telephony.

As far as plastic surgery is concerned, they can carry out all procedures but specialise in breast surgery, facial and head contouring, and body contouring.

For patients wanting gender reassignment (male-to-female), a letter is required from a medical doctor or a psychologist stating that the person is a suitable candidate for reassignment. Anyone who is HIV positive is asked to pay an extra 30 per cent of the charge because of the risk to hospital personnel. GR patients must be at least 18 years old and those under 20 will require permission from parents. They must complete a health check within three months of surgery and discontinue any hormone treatment at least 14 days prior to admission. The hospital stay is seven to ten days and the neo vagina created should be able to function within six weeks. Costs should be discussed with Phuket Health and Travel

The company also provides dental treatment. Here are some examples of charges:

Tooth whitening with laser:	£165
Porcelain veneer:	£110
Root canal treatment (one root):	£40–55
Ceramic crown:	£110
Implant:	£800–1,100
Complete dentures:	£180–205

At the time of writing, the company was offering special offers on health checks. For example:

Basic programme consisting of:

1 Physical examination by a doctor
2 Complete blood count (CBC)
3 Blood sugar level testing for diabetes (FBS)
4 Liver function test
   – SGPT
   – Alkaline Phosphatase
5 Kidney function test
   – Creatinine
   – BUN
6 Uric Acid
7 Lipid profile
   – Total cholesterol
   – Triglyceride
   – HDL cholesterol
   – LDL cholesterol
8 Urine examination (UA)

9   Stool examination
10 Chest X-ray
11 Electrocardiogram (EKG)
Cost: £40

There are also bigger health-check packages, which add hepatitis profiles and a mammogram test plus much more for women, and a prostate-cancer test and banks of other tests for men. They are aimed at the over-60s and cost from £170 to £210. They can also arrange for MRI scanning and dialysis treatment for kidney patients.

The majority of treatments are carried out at Bangkok Phuket Hospital, which has 44 full-time specialists and 50 consulting physicians in all areas. It has a certificate from the Quality Science Universal Company based in Singapore and was opened in 1995. There are 144 single rooms with en-suite bathrooms and 97 registered nurses.

Package deals including accommodation can also be arranged for many of the specialities and procedures, especially orthopaedic surgery such as hip and knee replacements, which gives the patient time to recover while staying on Patong Beach.

Here is an example for someone who might want double eyelid surgery to get rid of those bags with a six-night stay at Patong:

Day 1: Met at Phuket International Airport and transferred to the accommodation. Physical check-up at

Bangkok Phuket Hospital. Dinner and a show at Phuket Fantasea.

Day 2: Have double-eyelid surgery.
Leisure time at accommodation.
Day 3: Relax at accommodation or go for
a walk near by.
Day 4: Day at leisure on the beach at location
of hotel.
Day 5: A full-day Phuket explorer with lunch.
Day 6: Day at leisure.
Day 7: Follow-up procedure and stitch removal at
Bangkok Phuket Hospital. Transfer to Phuket
International Airport.
Prices start from £627, depending on
accommodation.

Tooth-whitening treatment with three nights' accommodation at Patong, a dinner and show, a sea-cave canoe tour plus all transfers costs from £307. Return flights from the UK are not included in any of the treatment or package prices.

Ferdia O'Dowd from Dublin, Ireland, went to the Bangkok Phuket Hospital in Phuket, Thailand, for dental work.

He says, 'When I was leaving – with two teeth perfectly restored – members of the hospital's international department persuaded me to take part in their 'Senior Executive Health Check Programme'. It showed strong evidence of a heart problem – of which I knew nothing.

'Three hours later I was in theatre watching on a TV monitor as dye was blown into my heart. After this was over, the senior guy came (complete with his own hand-drawn sketch) and showed me that one of the lower arteries had serious disease, and that they proposed treatment for the following day, using a balloon to blow the artery out to normal size and then inserting a metal 'stent' to keep the artery open permanently.

'I had walked into one of the best private hospitals in Southeast Asia and one of only two in Thailand outside Bangkok with a heart department capable of doing this very high-tech work (they also perform open-heart surgery). If you, like me, are a middle-aged man and have not had a full physical check-up for some years (if ever), consider taking the opportunity.'

RESTORED BEAUTY GETAWAYS
(www.restoredbeauty.com)
PO Box 581, Inglewood WA 6932, Australia
Tel: +61 8 9371 7142 Fax: +61 8 9371 6202
Email: info@restoredbeauty.com
Aimed mainly at the Australian medical tourist, this is an agent for the Bangkok Pattaya Hospital but has representatives in Thailand who offer a personal pick-up service from the airport and transfers, as well as taking care of all hospital procedures. All the usual cosmetic-surgery treatments are available as well as promotional health-check packages.

AESTHETIC SURGERY CENTER

(http://www.mtfsurgery.com)

340 Ladpraw 94, Sriwara Rd, Wangtonglang, Bangkok 10310

Tel: +66 2 559 0155 Fax: +66 2 559 2808

Email: info@mtfsurgery.com

The centre undertakes gender reassignment, however, it warns patients that it is not a cure for transsexualism but is more successful for people already enjoying a life in their chosen gender role. The centre, which also specialises in cosmetic surgery, can also arrange hotel reservations, tourist information and transportation.

The favoured hotel is the Maxx Hotel Bangkok, located at the heart of the new business centre of Bangkok next to Royal City Avenue, one of the longest shopping avenues in Asia. Special room rates for the hotel, which has a swimming pool, bar, cocktail lounge, health club, coffee shop, tennis courts and golf course, have been negotiated with standard rooms starting from as little as £14 a night.

Here are some prices for anyone wanting gender reassignment:

Penile skin inversion plus skin graft: $7,000 (£3,900)

One stage sigmoid colon: $8,000 (£4,450)

Second stage sigmoid colon: $6,600 (£3,670)

Cosmetic and functional correction: $2,200–3,300 (£1,230–1,840)

Bilateral orchiectomy: $2,200 (£1,230)

The centre also does cut-price package deals for sex-change patients who want to combine their procedures with cosmetic surgery. Their top package of penile skin inversion plus scrotal skin graft, with Adam's apple shaving, forehead and chin contouring and augmentation mammoplasty costs $12,000 (£6,700) against a usual cost of $14,150 (£7,900).

If clients just want cosmetic surgery, some costs for the most popular procedures are as follows:

Full facelift: $4,000 (£2,350)
Forehead lift: $2,200 (£1,300)
Cheekbone contouring: $2,200 (£1,300)
Jaw reduction: $2,750 (£1,620)
Breast augmentation: $2,500 (£1,470)
Breast reduction: $3,500 (£2,058)
Liposuction: $1,650 (£970)
Hair transplantation: $3,000 (£1,764)
Rhinoplasty: $1,650–2,750 (£970–1,620)

SAMUI CLINIC
(http://sexchangeasia.com)
Box 109, Nathon Post Office,
Koh Samui 84140, Thailand
Tel: +66 1 923 907 Fax: +66 77 422 566
Email: nickconnor4@aol.com
A sex-change clinic located on the tropical island of Koh Sumai, which boasts savings of up to 100 per cent compared with other countries. They advise patients to plan on being in Thailand for at least two to three

weeks, and use a Brandon Group Hospital located in Surat Thani on Koh Sumai. Patients spend two days in preparation and five days in hospital.

The clinic appears to concentrate on male-to-female reassignment, with costs as follows:

Vaginoplasty: $5,000 (£2,900)
Breast augmentation with prosthesis: $2,200 (£1,290)
Adam's apple shaving: $900 (£520)

Thailand is South-East Asia's biggest tourist destination thanks mainly to the fact that there is something for everyone, from the bustling shopping of Bangkok to the mountains of Mae Hong Son and the island resorts in the Andaman Sea. Whether it's culture or cuisine you want, you can get it in Thailand.

The country has a tropical climate, with summer from March to May, the rainy season from June to September and cool from October to February. English is widely understood, especially in Bangkok. The most popular places to visit are the capital – where skyscrapers mingle with temples and street markets to give the place a vibrancy that can spin your head around – and the beautiful island of Phuket, which picked itself up after the tsunami in double-quick time. Phuket has an excellent nightlife, great beaches, diving and fishing.

Chiang Mai, right up in the north, is a world away from Bangkok. Here, historic temples and incredible mountain scenery with wild elephants vie for attention – but there are still five-star hotels!

Koh Sumai is the third largest Thai island and had been a secret for years. Much more laid-back than Phuket, it's a place to chill.

FARES

Return economy fares to Phuket can start at around £500 depending on the carrier used, but can go up to £750 if you want to travel with British Airways. Flights to Bangkok are cheaper and if you shop around you can get a flight as low as £400–450.

> All private hospital rooms in Thailand have a full-length couch. Here, a relative or friend can sleep free of charge if they wish to stay with the patient instead of returning to their hotel room.

TUNISIA

OFFICIAL NAME: Tunisian Republic
AREA: 163,610 square kilometres (63,170 square miles)
POPULATION: 10,074,951
LANGUAGE: Arabic
CAPITAL: Tunis
TIME ZONE: Central European Time (GMT +1)
DISTANCE: London to Tunis = 1,830 kilometres
(1,137 miles)

As anyone who has holidayed there will know, Tunisia boasts some of the best white sandy beaches and clear water in the Mediterranean. What is more, its French colonial tradition means it is a unique crossroads between Europe and North Africa, where Arabic women stroll and shop in the famous souks of Tunis while wearing chic, Western-style clothing.

In recent years, the country's economy has been revitalised with an ever-growing middle class and a plethora of private clinics and hospitals springing up. It is no wonder, then, that Tunisia has started to see itself as a medical-tourist destination offering treatment at very affordable prices, all within a two-and-a-half-hour flight of the UK.

COSMETICA TRAVEL
www.cosmeticatravel.com

Immeuble Miniar, Rue des Lacs de Mazurie, Apt 1,
B1 Les Berges du Lac, 1053 Tunis
Tel: +216 71 965 265 Fax: +216 71 965 197
Email: contact@cosmeticatravel.com

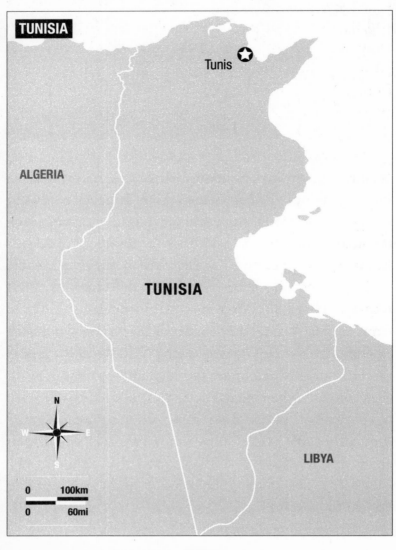

Usually specialise in cosmetic and dental surgery with all-inclusive trips to Tunisia, but can also arrange for orthopaedic surgery and ophthalmic surgery. The company says they deal with the best cosmetic surgeons in the country, all of whom have been trained abroad and speak English. In January 2005, the company was featured on *GMTV*, with Lorraine Kelly discussing the growth of medical tourism in Tunisia. It had testimony from an English woman, who had undergone breast augmentation and liposuction there and was happy with the results.

The surgeons used are registered with the Tunisian Medical Council and operate in top private clinics. All the small clinics offer a personal service and are only 15 minutes away from the capital's airport and hotels. They are the Alyssa Clinic, La Soukra Clinic, Berges du Lac Clinic, El Amen Clinic and La Marsa Clinic.

Hotel accommodation is at the five-star Corinthia Khamsa Hotel in the upmarket northern suburb of Gammarth, on a sandy beach and 20 minutes from the airport. It has 280 rooms and 29 suites, indoor and outdoor swimming pools, tennis courts, fitness centre, Turkish bath and a beach with parasols.

The prices for treatment include all hospital and surgical charges plus pre- and post-operation consultant's charges, any prostheses needed and five nights at the Corinthia Khamsa Hotel on a half-board basis. They do not include return flights from the UK to Tunis.

Here are examples of some of the prices:

COSMETIC

Forehead lift: €2,700 (£1,890)

Full facelift: €3,500 (£2,450)

Otoplasty: €1,200 (£840)

Rhinoplasty: €1,800 (£1,260)

Hair transplants: €1,900 (£1,330)

Breast augmentation: €2,500 (£1,750)

Breast reduction: €2,700 (£1,890)

Breast uplift: €2,500 (£1,750)

Tummy tuck: €2,700 (£1,890)

Liposuction (one or two areas): €2,000 (£1,400)

Eyelids (four): €1,700 (£1,190)

Eyelids (two – upper and lower): €1,500 (£1,000)

DENTAL

Ceramic crown: €350 (£240)

Metal crown: €226 (£160)

Bridge: €350 (£240)

One implant: €1,250 (£860)

Teeth whitening: €450 (£310)

The beaches around the capital – the Bay of Tunis – are not the best in Tunisia and certainly not as good as further south in places like Mahdia. But there is a lot to see in Tunis, which has developed into one of the best cities in North Africa.

Although Carthage may seem to be a bit of a disappointment because of the lack of really big ruins, a wander around this suburban area on the coast can be quite uplifting, thanks to the open spaces between those ruins that are left and the strange tranquillity of a place that is quite upmarket. The stops on the tiny train up the coast have evocative names like Hannibal, Byrsa and Salammbo.

The Roman mosaics in the city's Le Bardo museum are well worth seeing, and the souks in the Tunis medina are endlessly fascinating with their mix of tourist kitsch, small coffee shops, mosques and everyday goods for sale from sandals to perfume and sunglasses to henna. The well-laid-out French 'new town', with its wide main boulevard, is great for people-watching while it has some excellent and cheap restaurants down its side streets.

Cosmetica Travel can arrange for any excursions a client might like to take either before or after treatment, including spa cures, a visit to the pretty hillside village of Sidi Bou Said, Carthage, the medina and the museum as well as a trip to the country's most famous seaside resort of Hammamet. A three-day excursion to the Sahara Desert can also be enjoyed before treatment.

FARES
Direct economy return flights to Tunis by either Tunis Air or British Airways can be found for around £200–250 at a bucket shop, depending on the time of year you wish to fly. Cosmetica Travel has also done a deal with Tunis Air. On presentation of a letter confirming your surgery appointment and signed by the director of Cosmetica Travel, you will be able to enjoy a special tariff on the purchase of an open return ticket.

Although the price of your medical treatment will be fixed, just about everything else in Tunisia can be bargained for – and nowhere better than in the souks of Tunis, some of the best markets in the Arab world. Don't be frightened to start with a derisory offer. As a rule of thumb begin with a quarter or a fifth of the price asked.

TURKEY

OFFICIAL NAME: Republic of Turkey
AREA: 780,580 square kilometres (301,384 square miles)
POPULATION: 69,660,559
LANGUAGE: Turkish (official), Kurdish
CAPITAL: Ankara
TIME ZONE: Eastern European Time (GMT +2)
DISTANCE: London to Istanbul = 2,510 kilometres
(1,560 miles)

Turkey is fast becoming a favourite playground for British holidaymakers, taking over from the traditional love of Spain. And it's not hard to see why. Prices in Spain have risen steeply since the introduction of the euro, while Turkey is still relatively cheap. And the same goes for its medical infrastructure, where prices are way down on those in Western Europe. No wonder, then, that as the country's travel tourism starts to boom its medical tourism is also beginning to take off.

MEDTRAVEL TURKEY
(www.medtravelturkey.com/)
Ali Rîza Gürcan Caddesi, 30/21 Alparslan, Merkezi Merter, Istanbul, Turkey
Tel: +90 212 481 67 32 Fax: +90 212 481 67 36
Email: info@medtravelturkey.com
Set up to deal with medical tourists wanting dental,

283

cosmetic, eye and infertility treatment. They offer a package deal, which includes a hotel in Istanbul, or you can elect to have treatment only.

You can choose between a four- or five-star hotel, both of which are in Istanbul city centre, and a single room, or a double room if a relative or friend is accompanying you. The excellent website has prices for all procedures and package deals, and a reservation form. The package deals include airport transfers and transfers to the hospital, as well as hotel accommodation on a bed and breakfast basis and all treatment costs.

Here are some examples of a four-star hotel package deal on a double-room basis with the total nights of hotel accommodation. Return flights to Istanbul are not included:

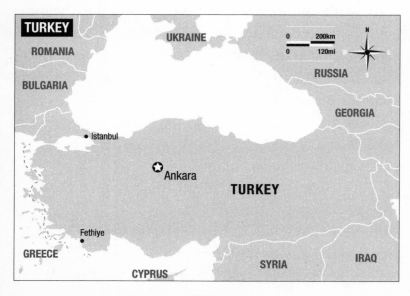

TURKEY

LASIK eye surgery:	€ 1,250 (£834)	4 nights

COSMETIC

Nose surgery:	€ 3,750 (£2,500)	10 nights
Breast enlargement:	€ 4,875 (£3,250)	10 nights
Breast reduction:	€ 4,875 (£3,250)	10 nights
Breast lift:	€ 4,575 (£3,050)	10 nights
Liposuction (one or two parts):	€ 2,920 (£1,947)	7 nights
Hair implants:	€ 3,270 (£2,180)	5 nights
Facelift:	€ 6,750 (£4,500)	10 nights
Tummy tuck:	€ 5,395 (£3,597)	14 nights
Gynaecomastia:	€ 3,450 (£2,300)	7 nights
Ear surgery:	€ 2,875 (£2,875)	5 nights
Upper and lower eyelid surgery:	€ 3,225 (£2,150)	6 nights

FERTILITY

IVF – ICSI:	€ 3,985 (£2,660)	17 nights
IUI – Inseminations:	€ 1,850 (£1,234)	7 nights
Second attempt and more:	€ 3,375 (£2,250)	17 nights

DENTAL

Teeth bleaching:	€ 920 (£614)	2 nights
Porcelain implant:	€ 1,850 (£1,234)	4 nights
Complete prostheses:	€ 3,850 (£2,567)	7 nights

INTERNATIONAL HEALTH TOURISM
Cumhuriyet Cad Beler Palas No 47/2, Kat: 4 D: 16
Taksim, Istanbul
Tel: +90 212 237 84 64 Fax: +90 212 327 84 52

Email: nihan@internationalhealthtourism.com

A similar operation to Medtravel Turkey, offering four- or five-star hotel accommodation in Istanbul as a package deal with cosmetic, dental and eye surgery. All hospital and airport transfers are included in the price, along with all treatment costs and even a half-day city tour. Examples of four-star doubles with total nights' hotel accommodation are:

COSMETIC

Hair implants:	€3,314 (£2,210)	10 nights
Breast surgery:	€5,108 (£3,405)	14 nights
Liposuction:	€3,709 (£2,473)	7 nights
Nose surgery:	€3,682 (£2,455)	10 nights

OTHER

LASIK eye surgery:	€1,268 (£845)	4 nights

DENTAL IN TURKEY

(www.dentalinturkey.com/)

No 178/7 Fetip Merkezi Gunlukbasi, Fethiye

Tel: +90 252 613 66 36 Fax: +90 542 644 81 57

Email: info@dentalinturkey.com

A small dental practice in the western Mediterranean coastal resort of Fethiye, this is ideal for anyone wanting to combine treatment with a holiday in the town, or other Turquoise Coast resorts such as Calis and Oludeniz. All staff speak English.

The practice will pick you up from your hotel and take you to and from the clinic. They can also arrange your hotel accommodation, if you wish, with transfers to and from the airport.

They say, 'All you need to do is drop us an email telling us what you want doing, send us a panoramic X-ray of your teeth by post and we'll give you a quote on accommodation and treatment.

'We'll work out a complete programme for you, which will include day trips out (optional), relaxation time and of course a treatment schedule.'

Here are a few prices, for treatment only:

Porcelain crown: £75
Ceramic crown: £130
Three tooth bridge: £200–400
Nine tooth bridge: £500–1,200
Tooth implant including top structure: £550–1,000

FARES

Flights to Istanbul vary according to the time of the year and how late you leave it until you book. Expect to pay between £140 and £200 for an economy return.

Remember to pack your diarrhoea tablets, as Turkey has a reputation for the 'Ottoman Revenge', especially outside the tourist resorts. And be careful not to overeat. In fact you should undereat at the beginning of your stay to allow your digestive system to become familiar with local food.

INDEX